FEELGOOD FOODS

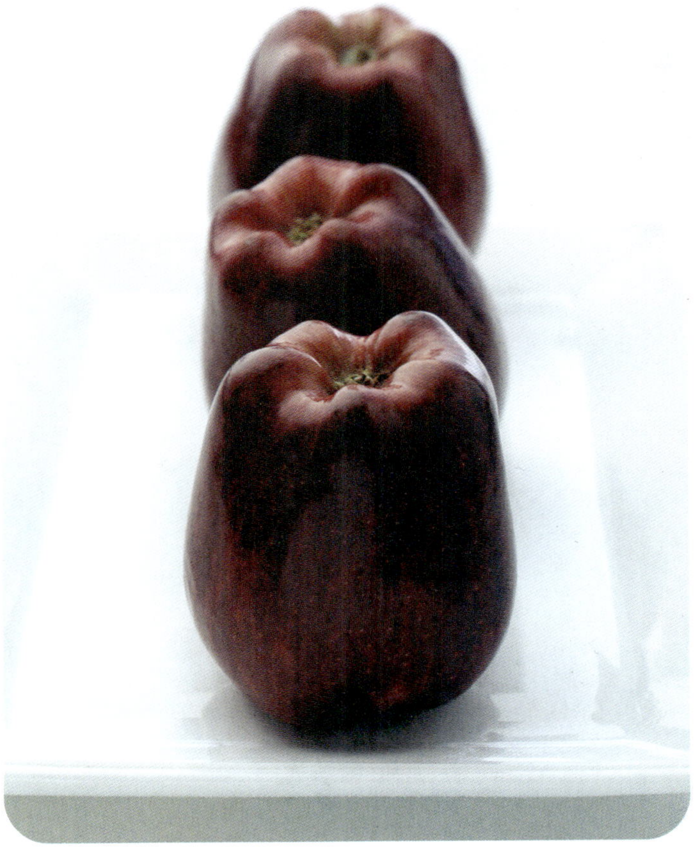

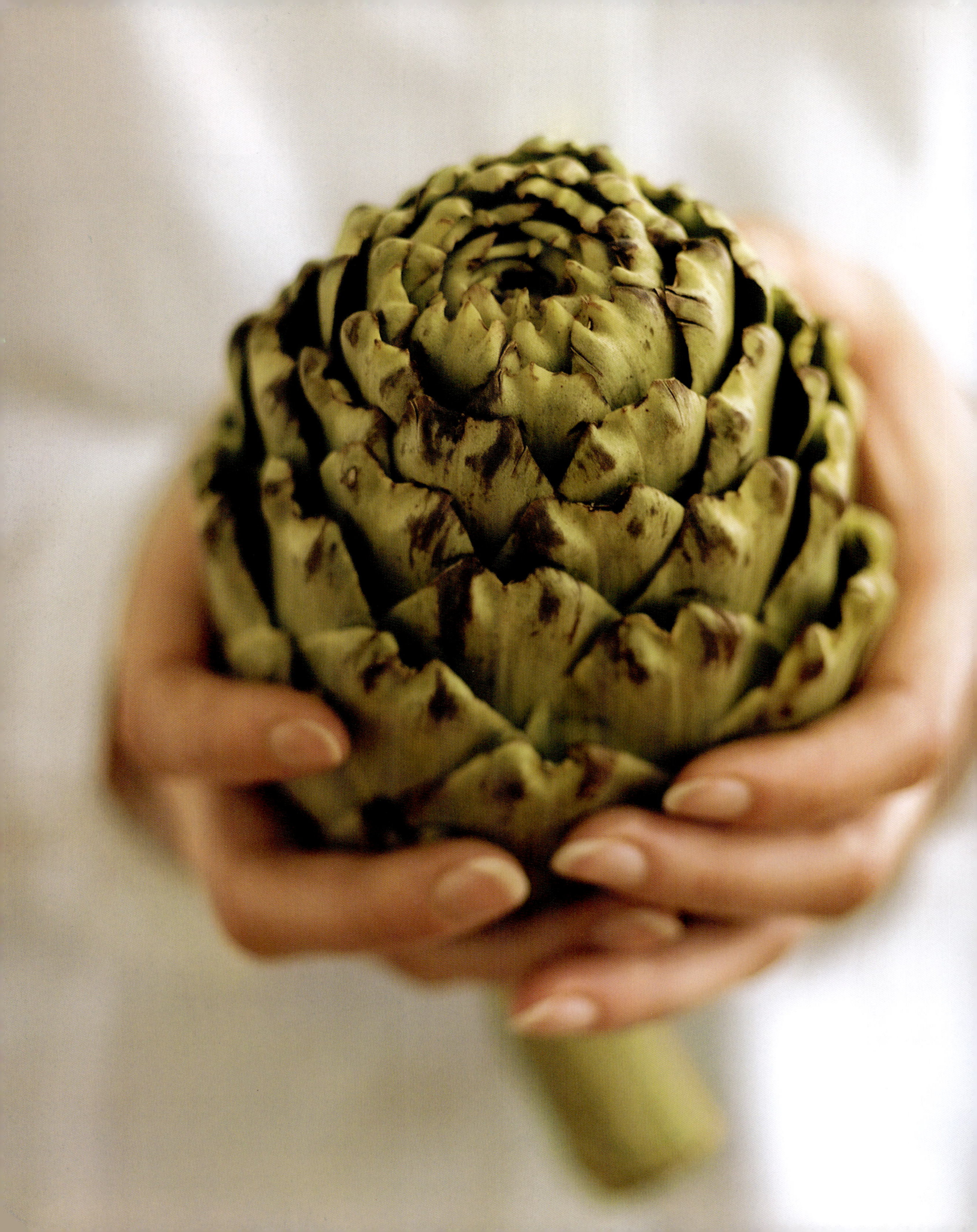

NATALIE SAVONA

FEELGOOD FOODS

FOODS AND RECIPES FOR A HEALTHY MIND

dbp

DUNCAN BAIRD PUBLISHERS

LONDON

FEEL GOOD FOODS
Natalie Savona

Conceived, created, and designed by Duncan Baird Publishers Ltd
Sixth Floor
Castle House
75–76 Wells Street
London W1T 3QH

Managing Editor: Judy Barratt
Editor: Joanne Clay
Managing Designer: Manisha Patel
Commissioned Photography: William Lingwood
Photography Assistant: Emma Bentham-Wood
Stylists: David Morgan, Helen Trent

British Library Cataloging-in-Publication Data:
A CIP record for this book is available from the British Library

ISBN: 1-904292-33-X

10 9 8 7 6 5 4 3 2 1

Typeset in Helvetica Neue
Color reproduction by Scanhouse, Malaysia
Printed and bound in Singapore by Imago

PUBLISHER'S NOTE: *Feel Good Foods* is not intended as a replacement for professional medical treatment and advice. The publishers and authors cannot accept responsibility for any damage incurred as a result of any of the therapeutic methods contained in this work. If you are suffering from a medical condition and are unsure of the suitability of any of the therapeutic methods or food supplements mentioned in this book, or if you are pregnant, it is advisable to consult a medical practitioner. Essential oils must be diluted in a base oil before use. They should not be taken internally and are for adult use only. The detox program on pages 36–7 should be avoided by children, elderly people, and women who are pregnant or breast feeding.

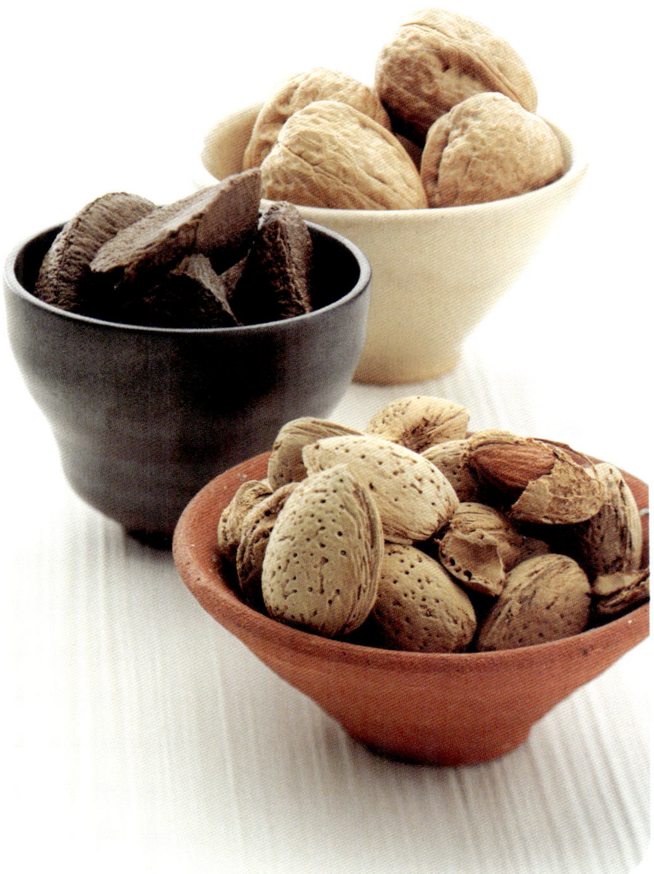

This book is for anyone interested in choosing their food and lifestyle for a peaceful mind and abundant physical energy.

contents

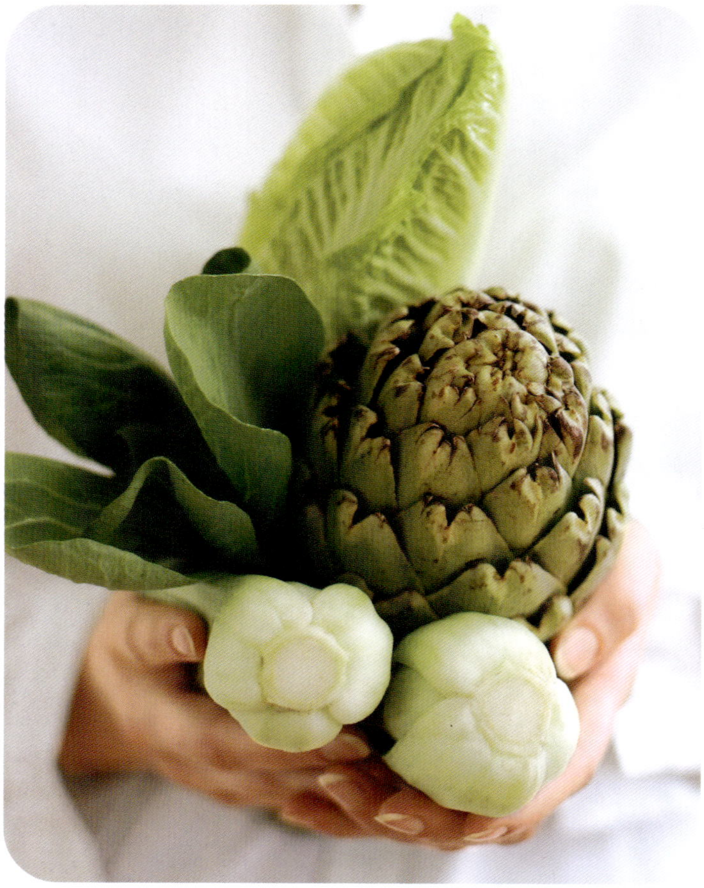

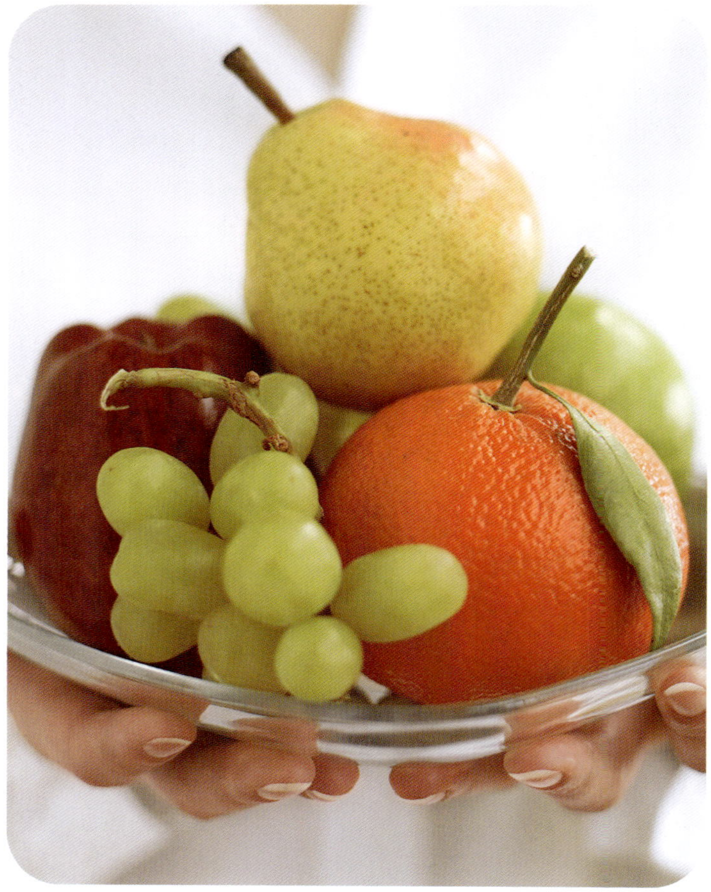

Introduction 8

CHAPTER 1

THE PHYSIOLOGY OF MELANCHOLY 10

Blood-Sugar Balance 12

The Stress Response 18

Nutrient Supplies 22

Healthy Fats 26

Waste Disposal 30

Food Sensitivity 38

CHAPTER 2

MOOD'S MANY GUISES 40

How to Use This Chapter 42

Energy Deficit 44

Premenstrual Problems 48

Winter Woes: SAD 52

Sleepless Nights 54

Binge Eating 58

Brain Slow-Down 62

Depression 66

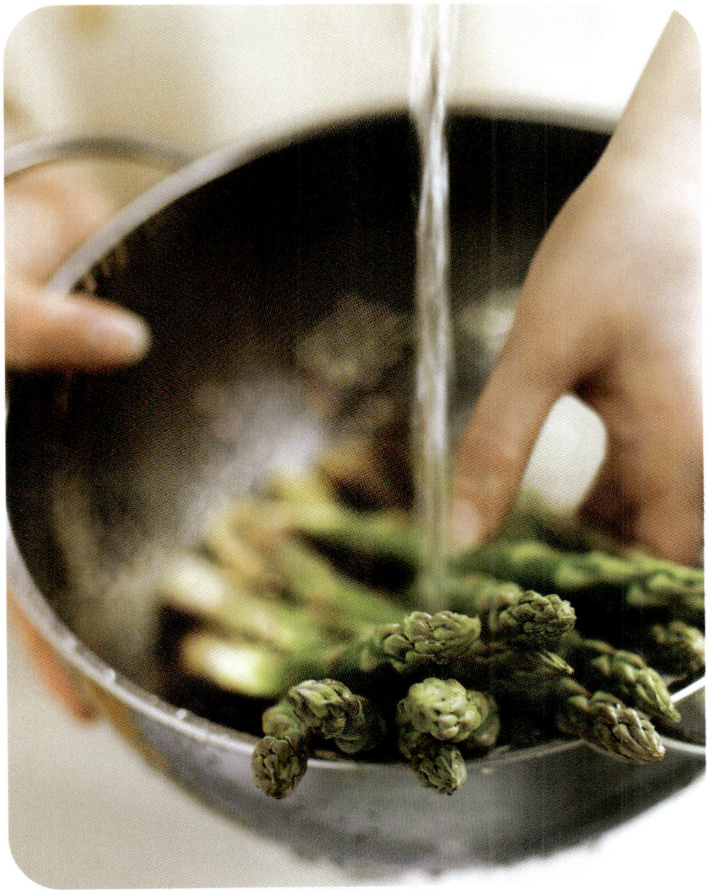

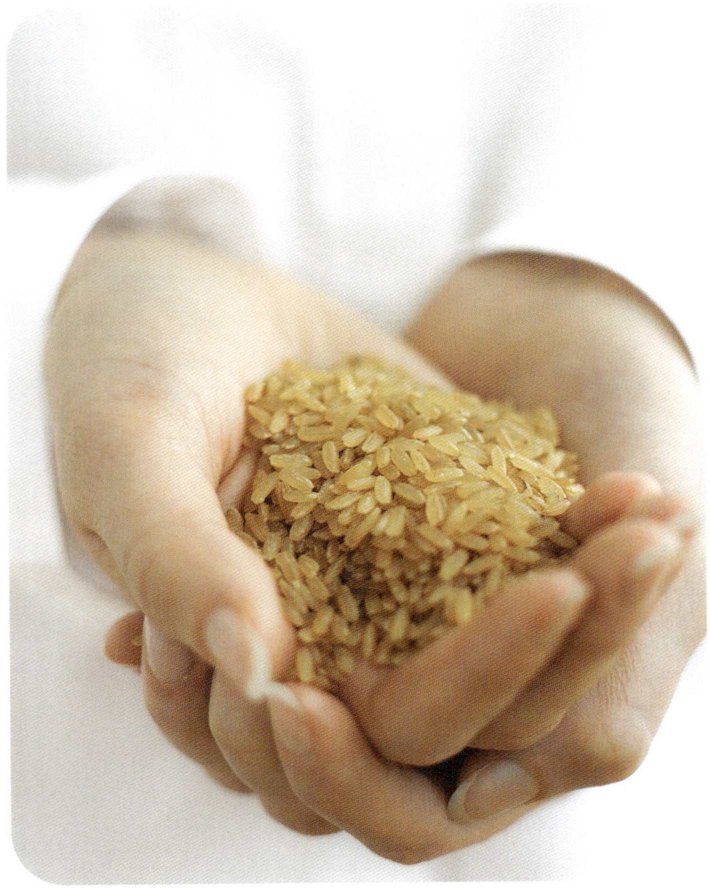

CHAPTER 3

FEEL GOOD FOOD **72**

Feel Good Diet 74

Pantry 78

Feel Good Recipes: Breakfasts 80

Starters and Lunches 84

Soups 94

Main Meals 100

Side Dishes, Side Salads 114

Desserts 118

Snacks 124

CHAPTER 4

THE WHOLE PICTURE **126**

Feel Good Supplements 128

Nutrients and Rich Food Sources 130

Feel Good Strategies 132

Glossary 136

Further Reading 138

Useful Addresses 139

Index 140

Acknowledgments 144

introduction

In February 1995 I ate nothing for two weeks. Strangely, it was that period of eating nothing that eventually led to my work with food. I had found myself on a beach in Thailand, fasting with a group of like-minded souls. That is, we were like-minded in as much as we were all aiming at cleansing and regenerating our bodies and minds, but otherwise we were as unalike as could be. There was an ex-junkie call girl from New Zealand, a psychotherapist from the United States, a back-packer from England, and me, a lapsed journalist who had spent the previous 18 months living in Bangkok, all supervized by an ex-television newscaster from Canada.

For those two weeks, all that passed my mouth was water, coconut water, and a sludgy mixture of herbs and clay. I can honestly say I felt fantastic—no, it was not delirium, and yes, it was helped by the idyllic Thai-beach setting, the daily yoga, and swimming in the ocean. Now, in case you are about to put this book down, thinking that I am a confirmed, extreme health nut, about to recommend that you do as I did, let it be known that I have just drained a cup of coffee and have a bottle of good red wine sitting by my front door to take to dinner at a friend's tonight, where I shall eat whatever is put in front of me, be that chips and cheesecake or salad and sunflower seeds.

Living in Bangkok was a fascinating experience, but one that left me exhausted and depressed. Exhausted to the extent that I would stand, hawk-eyed on a packed bus home from work, desperate to spot a twitch that would indicate the next person to vacate a seat. Depressed to the extent that I gave up my job and spent a considerable amount of time lying around on cushions, crying. The potential triggers for what was described by one healthcare practitioner as my "chronic fatigue" were manifold and mysterious: a difficult relationship leading to panic attacks and insomnia, living in a polluted city, reliance on coffee, perhaps even too many margaritas on Friday nights ... who knows? What I do know is that I felt immeasurably better after fasting for two weeks, which led me to investigate what may have been going on inside me.

After trying various strategies in a bid to rediscover my lively and enthusiastic self, I started studying nutrition formally. I can certainly say that a combination of factors have helped restore my physical and emotional health, but the foundation for them all is now what I eat and drink each day. At nutrition college, I wrote a dissertation on the use of nutritional strategies in dealing with depression—a project which went on to form the germ of this book. What follows is, in a way, wisdom that I gained on my personal journey to restore balance in my body and mind.

Research study after research study finds that too many people in Western society are tired and down. Although modern life is supposedly becoming ever more convenient and less labor-intensive, many of us are simply exhausted, and poor mental health is rapidly becoming a significant concern. A report published in 2001 found that seven percent of adults in the United States, and nearly 10 percent in the United Kingdom, France, Germany, Italy, and Spain were suffering from major depression. The number of people who constantly felt "low" was found to be many times higher than that. The World Health Organization predicts that depression is poised to move up to ranking second as the most common disorder in the world after heart disease by 2020. Such a scenario is not just a personal tragedy for the sufferer and his or her family but also a considerable burden on healthcare systems.

However, energy and mood problems do not have to be an inevitable part of modern life. You can feel good. Being healthy does not just mean being free from classifiable disease: It means being able to live a full life. Our body systems do not function in isolation as modern medicine, with its numerous "specialities," would have us believe—we are complex creatures, sensitive to everything happening around us and within us. To separate our mood and energy levels from other goings-on in our bodies is like expecting a television to produce a clear picture no matter where the aerial is, no matter whether it is switched on, no matter whether every single part of the TV is in working order. Where your emotional and physical health are concerned, a nutritional approach can help ensure that all parts of the body are working as optimally as possible and in harmony with one another.

The information on the following pages is aimed at inspiring you to believe that you do have the power to maintain your energy and moods at optimum levels. Although our wellbeing is, of course, influenced by many factors—including the genes we are born with, the way we react to life events, and the environment in which we live—we are also chemical beings who can, to a certain degree, use the raw material with which we nourish our bodies to program our health. The information in this book is not designed to "treat" any serious psychological illnesses. Instead it is aimed at anyone who finds themselves constantly tired, down, suffering from poor sleep, premenstrual problems, binge eating, or unreliable brain power. Of course, the recommendations given may be a useful adjunct to the treatment of a medical condition that is a more serious form of any of these, under the guidance of a doctor.

My view is that the basics of eating for good moods are dictated by common sense: Eat food as close to its natural state as possible, eat a variety of foods, and relax and enjoy your meals. Few health concepts are as poorly consensual as the "balanced diet," but I consider the core element of a healthy-eating program to be just that—balance. Broccoli and brown rice are indeed healthy foods, but they alone will not sustain you. On the other hand, the occasional bar of chocolate or glass of red wine can be positively good for the soul.

You can use this book in several ways. You may like to read the whole of Chapter 1, The Physiology of Melancholy, to ascertain which underlying nutritional imbalances may be affecting your moods and learn about specific strategies for addressing those imbalances. You can then go to the section in Chapter 2, Mood's Many Guises, that resonates most with you. Here you will find practical solutions—largely nutritional, but also some lifestyle recommendations—that are designed to alleviate each mood-related condition. Alternatively, you may prefer to go straight to the relevant topic in Chapter 2, referring back to the more detailed information in Chapter 1 as it comes up.

In Chapter 3, Feel Good Food, you will find the nuts and bolts of what to actually put on your plate. From there, Chapter 4, The Whole Picture, describes a multifaceted approach, including the way you react to life events and the importance of keeping fit. The physical, biochemical aspects of mental wellbeing—although the main focus of this book—should be taken as just one part of the overall picture. As I always say, nutrition is a fundamental element in any healthy life, but it is only one of many.

Natalie

NATALIE SAVONA

AS MANY OF THE ANCIENT SAGES KNEW, BALANCE IS CRUCIAL IF YOU ARE TO MAINTAIN GOOD HEALTH. UNDERSTANDING EXACTLY HOW YOUR BODY SYSTEMS WORK IS AN IMPORTANT FIRST STEP IN REDRESSING ANY HIDDEN NUTRITIONAL IMBALANCES THAT MAY BE UNDERMINING THE MYRIAD PHYSICAL PROCESSES THAT GOVERN YOUR MOODS.

Feeling good in your body, mind, and soul calls for balance across all aspects of your life, including your diet. In this chapter, we examine how important body systems—such as blood-sugar balance, stress response, and detoxification—work, and explore why if any of your body's finely tuned mechanisms are even slightly off-key, symptoms such as low moods, insomnia, and cravings may result. We explore how your diet and lifestyle may be affecting your body functions—and therefore your moods and energy—and also discover ways of supporting the body systems that affect your mental health through a few straightforward dietary changes.

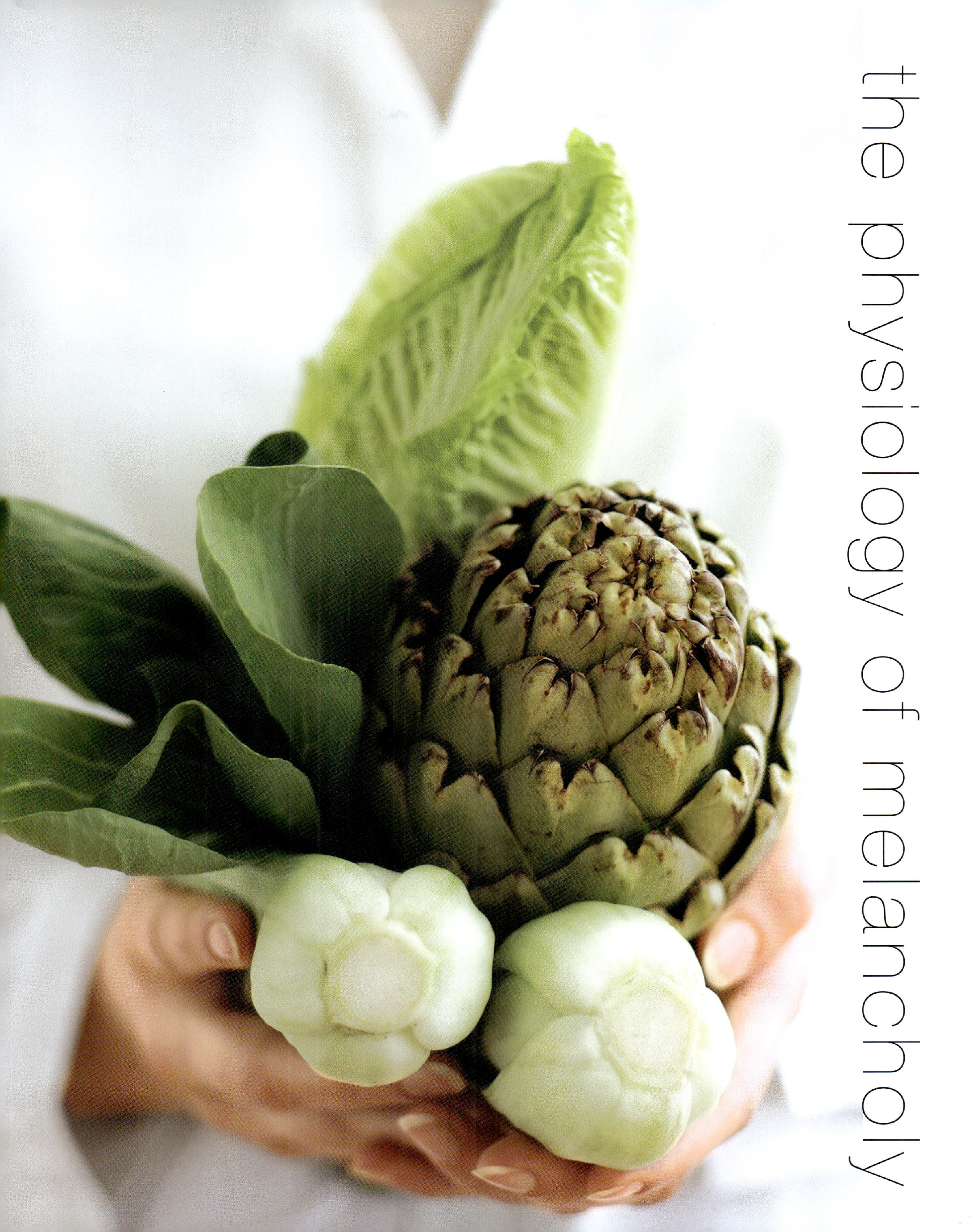

the physiology of melancholy

Do you suffer from recurrent dives in mood, concentration, and energy? Do you reach for a sugary snack or a cup of coffee to "pick you up," only to find you feel grumpy and exhausted again shortly afterward? By improving your eating habits, you can step off the "blood-sugar seesaw."

blood-sugar balance

On the list below, tick the symptoms that apply to you more or less daily:

- ☐ fatigue
- ☐ irritability
- ☐ cravings for sweet foods or drinks/coffee/tea/cigarettes
- ☐ a need for regular snacks
- ☐ lapses in mood/concentration/memory
- ☐ difficulty making decisions
- ☐ light-headedness
- ☐ sweating for no apparent reason
- ☐ "butterflies" in stomach for no apparent reason
- ☐ difficulty getting to sleep, or waking in the night
- ☐ headaches
- ☐ palpitations

If you ticked six or more of the above symptoms, you may be having difficulty keeping your blood sugar balanced, in which case you are probably familiar with the following scenario. At around three o'clock in the afternoon, you suddenly start to yawn, then your concentration goes, and a black cloud seems to move over the day. But never mind, you know how to cure all that—a cup of coffee, a cigarette, or a bar of chocolate soon does the trick, and you can get back to the task in hand ... until the next slump strikes.

Regular fluctuations in mood and energy are often linked to highs and lows in blood-sugar levels. These in turn are linked to the food we eat and drink, particularly sweet, sugary, and starchy foods. Such foods may temporarily fulfil a craving brought on by sudden tiredness and irritability, but they also cause our blood-sugar levels—and with them our energy and mood—to seesaw. Maintaining even blood-sugar levels is, therefore, one of the most crucial factors in improving our moods, and we will be returning to the subject throughout this chapter.

Brain fuel

If sugar is so harmful, why do we love it so much and even crave it? The brain requires a constant, optimum level of fuel and nutrients. One type of fuel is glucose—the smallest molecule of sugar, and the only form of sugar that the brain is able to accept as fuel. When we eat sugar, therefore, we are fulfilling the brain's need to receive a non-stop supply of glucose.

Pure sugar and sugar products are not the body's only sources of blood sugar. During digestion, carbohydrates—which are classified as "simple" or "complex" depending on their structure—can also be turned into sugars. Simple carbohydrates are those found in pure sugar, fruit sugar (fructose), and other sweeteners, such as honey or corn

BITE-SIZE SOLUTION

Breakfast's name comes from breaking your overnight fast—providing the body with fuel to get it going for the day. Skipping the most important meal of the day sets the scene for fluctuating blood-sugar levels. So always have breakfast, even if it's not as soon as you get up.

NUTRIENTS FOR BLOOD-SUGAR BALANCE

In order to maintain even blood-sugar levels, we need a full range of nutrients, which are best obtained from a varied, balanced diet. The following nutrients are particularly important:

Nutrient	Rich food sources
Protein	Dairy products, eggs, fish, meat, poultry, soy
Magnesium	Almonds, fish, green leafy vegetables, molasses, nuts, soybeans, sunflower seeds, wheatgerm
Chromium	Beef, brewer's yeast, chicken, eggs, fish, fruit, milk products, potatoes, whole grains
Vitamin B1	Beef kidney and liver, brewer's yeast, garbanzo beans, kidney beans, pork, rice bran, salmon, soybeans, sunflower seeds, wheatgerm, wholegrain wheat and rye
Vitamin B2	Almonds, brewer's yeast, cheese, chicken, wheatgerm
Vitamin B3	Beef liver, brewer's yeast, chicken, fish, sunflower seeds, turkey
Vitamin B5	Blue cheese, brewer's yeast, corn, eggs, lentils, liver, lobster, meats, peanuts, peas, soybeans, sunflower seeds, wheatgerm, whole grains
Vitamin C	Blackcurrants, broccoli, Brussels sprouts, cabbage, collard greens, grapefruit, green peppers, guava, lemons, oranges, papaya, potatoes, spinach, strawberries, tomatoes, watercress
Vanadium	Buckwheat, fish, mushrooms, parsley, shellfish, soy
Manganese	Barley, buckwheat, dried fruit, green leafy vegetables, nuts, oats, seaweed, whole grains

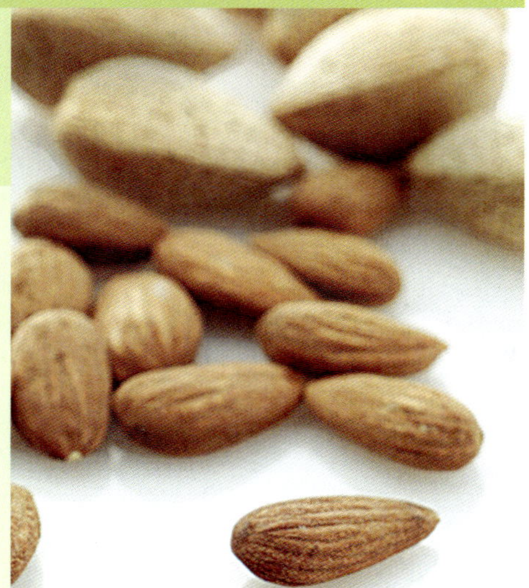

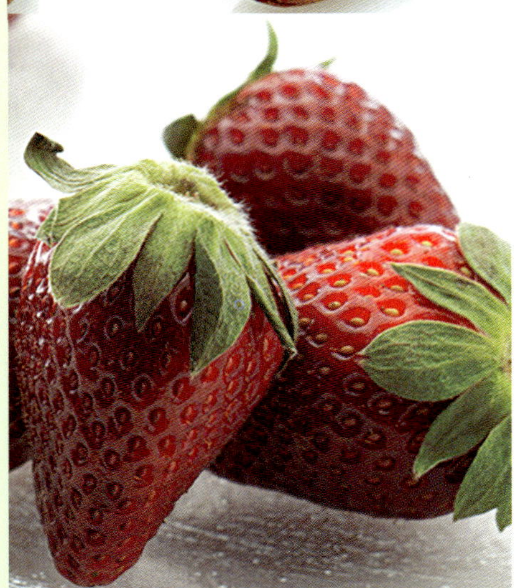

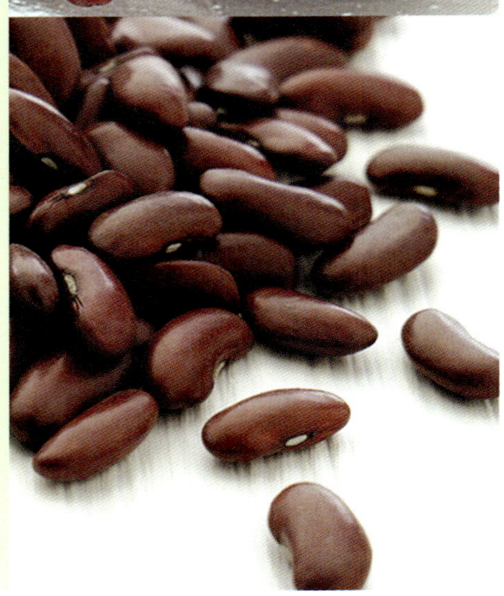

THE BLOOD-SUGAR SEESAW

The dotted yellow line in the diagram below represents normal, healthy fluctuations in blood-sugar levels that occur over a period of a few hours or a whole day, depending on your metabolism and diet. The red line represents undesirable extreme rises and falls in blood-sugar levels caused by a diet that throws the body's natural equilibrium out of kilter. If you notice that you are suddenly feeling tired and low, struggling to concentrate, and craving sweet, starchy food, you are probably experiencing a blood-sugar drop. A common reaction is to grab a sugary snack, which, combined with your body's own efforts to resolve the crisis (see page 15), causes blood-sugar levels to rise sharply. You may briefly feel better, but this sudden rise is quickly followed by another dramatic fall and the whole cyle begins again. This may occur twice during the day—mid-morning and mid-evening are often marked by drops in blood-sugar levels, especially if your breakfast and lunch are composed mainly of fast-releasing foods (see box, page 16)—or it may occur as often as once an hour, if you regularly snack on fast-releasing foods.

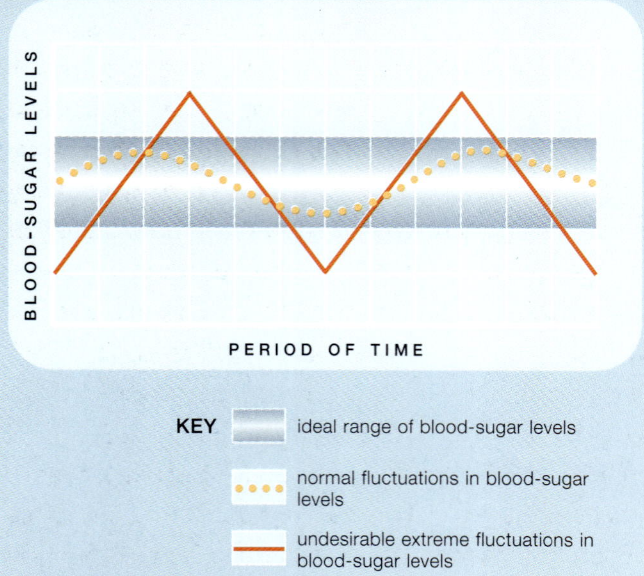

syrup. Complex carbohydrates, sometimes known as starches, are less sweet; they are broken down into glucose during digestion. Wheat (from which bread and pasta are made), rice, potatoes, and corn are all starches.

Starches that are combined with their naturally occurring fiber, such as brown rice, are digested more slowly and therefore provide the body with a more steady supply of glucose. So it is best to eat unrefined versions of starchy foods whenever possible and steer clear of processed foods, such as white bread.

The soar and slump

Our bodies are very carefully designed to maintain balance—otherwise known as homoeostasis—for example, no more or less water in the blood than is ideal, and no more or less of each given hormone. Blood sugar is no exception; in order to avoid potentially dangerous highs or lows, the body rapidly compensates for any changes in blood-sugar levels caused by food intake or a skipped meal.

Ideally, blood-sugar levels should fall slightly a few hours after a meal (thus triggering hunger) and rise as the digested meal passes into the bloodstream. However, many people's blood-sugar levels rise and fall dramatically throughout the day (see box, left). When blood sugar plummets, lethargy, sleepiness, irritability, and cravings set in, and perhaps even anxiety, palpitations, a headache, or light-headedness. These symptoms of low blood sugar prompt you to react—you have learned that a cup of coffee, a coke, a cigarette, or a bar of chocolate will give you the rapid fix you need. (Although coffee and cigarettes do not actually contain sugar, they stimulate the release of sugar stores in the body. Alcohol also raises blood-sugar levels only to send them plummeting again soon afterward.) Meanwhile, your body is busy taking its own urgent steps in order to get blood-sugar levels back within the ideal parameters. It rapidly releases stores of glucose and, at the same time, pumps out epinephrine to make sure the fuel gets around the body as quickly as possible.

However, in spite of all these efforts to raise blood-sugar levels, the relief from the slump lasts only for a short while. This is because, rather than raising blood-sugar levels to

WHAT IS YOUR DIET DOING TO YOUR BLOOD-SUGAR LEVELS?

One of the main reasons specific foods, certain eating patterns or missing meals affect the way you feel is that they have an impact on your blood-sugar levels. So what do they actually do to them?

Eating slow-releasing carbohydrates:	Blood sugar rises gradually over a few hours
Eating proteins with carbohydrates:	Blood sugar rises slowly over a few hours
Eating sugary foods/fast-releasing carbohydrates/sugary drinks:	Blood sugar rises within minutes, followed by a dramatic fall
Drinking caffeine:	Blood sugar rises rapidly, followed by a slump
Drinking alcohol:	Blood sugar rises and falls rapidly
Missing a meal:	Blood sugar drops. Missing breakfast can have dramatic effects because of the long gap between dinner today and lunch tomorrow

within the desirable parameters, our "quick fix" often pushes them beyond the ideal maximum. This is caused by a combination of the means we use—the chocolate, coffee, cigarette—and a by-now confused and over-reacting body. In order to deal with the sudden excess in blood sugar, the body sends out the hormone insulin, which helps to get glucose out of the blood and into the cells, where it is used for energy. The sudden release of too much insulin then sends blood-sugar levels crashing, leaving you craving yet another fix.

So how can you ensure that your body receives the sugar it needs without sending your blood-sugar levels into an exhausting and damaging soar-and-slump pattern?

Sugar surprises

An awareness of which foods perpetuate the blood-sugar seesaw allows you to be more in control of how you feel. As we have seen, sweet foods and stimulants make your blood sugar soar and consequently crash. They take with them your moods and energy—avoid them! However, it is not always obvious which foods contain sugar. It is easy to spot sugar in a cookie, a bar of chocolate, a piece of candy, a milkshake, or a doughnut. More insidious, though, are the hidden quantities of sugar contained in less obviously sweetened foods: bread, baked beans and other canned foods, fruit yogurt, fruit juices, breakfast cereals, ketchup and other sauces or dressings, as well as many convenience meals. You can see how the amount of sugar you are eating each day can easily creep up without you even realizing it. That is why it is a good idea to eat as many fresh, unprocessed foods as possible and to eat artificially sweetened foods only in small amounts. Check the backs of a few packets in supermarkets and see how high sugar comes on the list of ingredients.

If your blood-sugar levels are poorly balanced, even foods that are perfectly good for you, such as fruit juices or dried fruits, can create havoc in your body. Although natural, these foods are a very concentrated source of

GLYCAEMIC INDEX OF FOODS

Slow-releasing foods	Moderate-releasing	Fast-releasing	Very fast-releasing
fish/seafood	whole rye bread	all pasta	corn flakes
meat/poultry	oatmeal	oranges	cooked root vegetables
eggs	barley	peas	rice cakes
whole milk	basmati rice	baked beans	white bread
yogurt	buckwheat	potatoes	white and brown rice
cottage cheese	pitta bread	muesli	whole-kernel corn
soy/tofu	apples	popcorn	bananas
seeds/nuts	pears	wholewheat bread	dried fruit
tahini/houmous	grapes		apricots
green vegetables	peaches		mangoes
tomatoes	kiwi fruit		honey
mushrooms	carrots		
raw root vegetables	beets		
grapefruit	lentils		
plums	kidney beans		
	garbanzo beans		
	skimmed milk		
	low-fat yogurt		

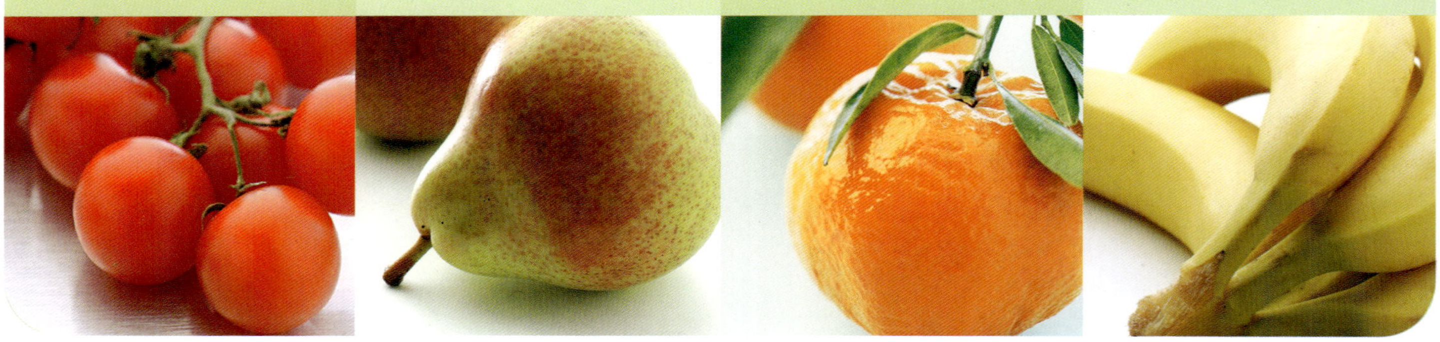

sugar. It is therefore best to dilute juices with 70 percent water and to eat dried fruits accompanied by some protein, such as a handful of nuts or a yogurt. (This slows down the rate at which the sugar contained in the fruit is released into your bloodstream.)

Eating to stabilize blood sugar

Your blood-sugar levels will be more stable if you eat regularly. Try not to skip breakfast (doing so means that by lunchtime the brain hasn't had a direct fuel delivery since dinner the night before) and never go more than four hours without food. If you found the symptoms listed at the beginning of this section very familiar, you will probably benefit from eating five or six small, regular meals throughout the day to keep your blood-sugar levels more even.

By choosing your food carefully, you can largely avoid steep rises in blood sugar. The glycaemic index (GI) has been devised as a method of defining food according to the speed at which it is digested and released into the bloodstream as glucose. The more fiber and protein (and fat) that are eaten alongside starchy or sugary foods, the more slowly those foods are digested and released as sugar into your system. Rice cakes, for example, are very fast releasing—they have a high GI score. However, when spread with houmous, which is rich in protein and fat, the GI is reduced. The table opposite gives the GI index of various common foods. For a more even release of glucose into the bloodstream, it is important to minimize your intake of high GI (fast-releasing) foods, and not to eat them on their own. When you eat higher GI foods, try to make sure that you combine them with low GI (slow-releasing) foods. For example:

- brown rice with stir-fried chicken and green vegetables
- a baked potato with tuna and salad
- a banana with a handful of pumpkin seeds
- pasta with clam sauce
- wholewheat toast with poached eggs
- muesli with soy milk or skimmed milk
- rice cakes with tahini/houmous

Fiber also plays an important role in the management of blood sugar. A fiber-rich meal is released as glucose into the bloodstream more slowly than one that is low in fiber, thereby raising blood-sugar levels gradually. The higher the fiber content of a food, the lower its GI score is likely to be.

Finally, certain nutrients, which are listed in the table on page 13, are known to help stabilize blood-sugar levels. If you are suffering from the symptoms listed on page 12, you may need to increase your intake of foods that are rich in these nutrients.

More on nutrients

In addition to eating low GI foods or slow-releasing combinations, certain nutrients can actually enhance the processes that regulate blood-sugar levels. Firstly, there is the mineral chromium, which appears to be involved in the insulin mechanism and therefore the regulating of sugar. Many people find it helpful to take 100 mcg of chromium at breakfast and lunch while they are working on balancing blood-sugar levels, because it can help reduce cravings.

Another mineral, magnesium, is essential for the conversion of glucose to the form it is stored as, and vice versa. Ideal forms of magnesium to use are magnesium ascorbate, actually a type of vitamin C that helps support the adrenal glands. These are likely to be working overtime if your blood-sugar levels are all over the place. Magnesium pantothenate is a combination of the mineral and vitamin B5, another good adrenal nutrient. The B vitamins, particularly B3, but also B1 and B2, are needed for the processing of sugar in the body—all are best taken as part of a multivitamin or B-complex tablet. The amino acid (protein building block) L-glutamine is another supplement that can help reduce carbohydrate or sugar cravings because it directly fuels the brain. Vanadium and manganese are minerals that are involved in the way the body deals with glucose. They are needed in only very small amounts, so are best included in a multivitamin blend rather than taken separately. A nutritionist will be able to help you work out which supplements would be best for your individual needs (see page 139).

GOOD-MOOD SUMMARY

To maximize blood-sugar balance:

- avoid coffee and tea
- avoid alcohol and cigarettes
- avoid sugar, foods containing sugar, honey, and dried and fresh fruits
- avoid refined foods (white bread, white rice, and so on), processed foods and fast foods (many contain "hidden" sugar, as well as chemicals and harmful fats)
- dilute fruit or vegetable juices with 70 percent water
- eat dried fruit with protein, such as natural yogurt, a handful of nuts, cottage cheese, and so on
- always eat breakfast
- eat small meals five or six times a day, and include some fiber- and protein-rich foods in each one
- see pages 80–125 for some healthy recipe, meal, and snack ideas
- consider taking nutritional supplements designed to support blood-sugar balance

Our bodies can handle stress of any sort for only a limited period of time. After that, the continued impact of stress results in low moods, a lack of energy, and an increased susceptibility to illness. Lifestyle and dietary changes can help optimize your body's ability to cope with stress.

the stress response

On the list below, tick the symptoms that apply to you more or less daily:

- ☐ easily angered or irritable
- ☐ feeling as though you can't cope
- ☐ exhaustion
- ☐ difficulty making decisions
- ☐ lacking motivation
- ☐ mood swings
- ☐ over-reacting to life's everyday stresses
- ☐ difficulty sleeping
- ☐ waking up anxious
- ☐ panic attacks
- ☐ feeling particularly groggy when you wake up in the morning

If you ticked six or more of the above symptoms, your body may be struggling to deal with stress.

Stress is not caused only by attempting to juggle too many responsibilities at once and striving to meet tight deadlines. The term stress encompasses anything that upsets the body's delicate equilibrium, whether it be emotional issues, lack of focus or satisfaction, poor diet, too much coffee or nicotine or alcohol, an ongoing illness, or depression.

Epinephrine rush

One of the first body mechanisms to fall prey to prolonged stress is blood-sugar balance (see pages 12–17). The body systems involved in trying to regulate seesawing blood-sugar levels can easily become exhausted. For example, when falling blood-sugar levels are making constant demands on them, the adrenal glands (there is one of these on top of each kidney) soon become burnt out, and are no longer able to perform their job efficiently. They adapt by rewiring the body into a "hyper" state, during which you may experience insomnia, anxiety, panic attacks, difficulty making decisions, and depression. Even if the original external stressor disappears, your body may well remain in alarm mode.

Epinephrine is one of the hormones produced by the adrenal glands. In times of danger, epinephrine plays a crucial role in our primitive "fight-or-flight response"—it helps blood carrying oxygen and sugar to be pumped around the body fast to feed the brain (so that you can make a quick decision) or the muscles (so that you can either fight or run away from the threat). These days, however, we rarely escape stress by fighting or fleeing. We often face ongoing stress factors that cause our bodies to release epinephrine almost constantly, leading to a vicious cycle of permanently taut muscles and pent-up tension.

BITE-SIZE SOLUTION

Drinking relaxing herbal teas, such as chamomile or borage (starflower), can often help to calm you down, whereas drinking coffee has the opposite effect, putting more pressure on your body's stress-response mechanisms.

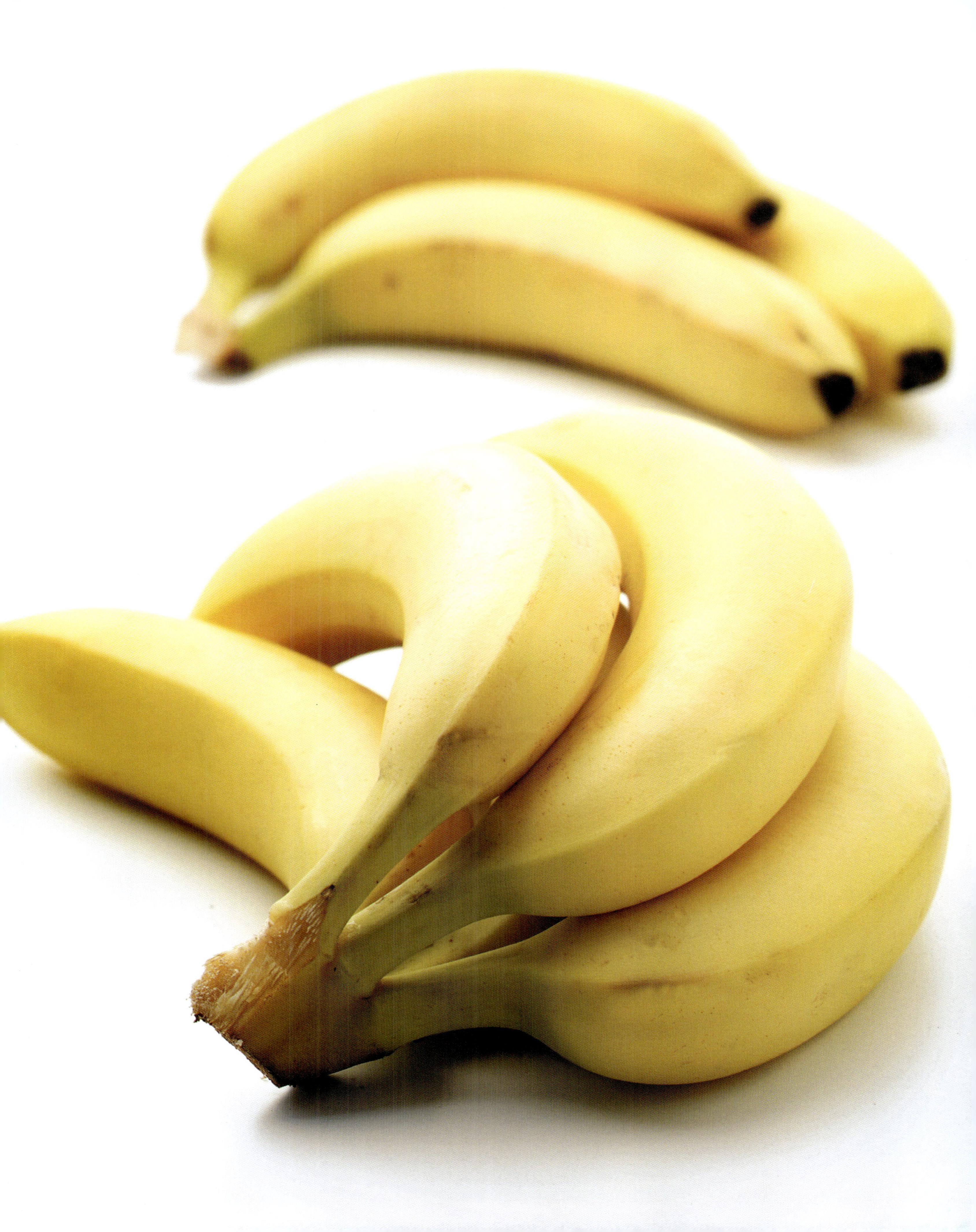

NUTRIENTS FOR HEALTHY STRESS RESPONSE

To optimize the body's response to stress, we need a full range of nutrients, which is best obtained from a varied, balanced diet. The following nutrients are particularly important:

Nutrient	Rich food sources
Protein	Dairy products, eggs, fish, meat, poultry, soy
Vitamin B3	Beef liver, brewer's yeast, chicken, fish, sunflower seeds, turkey
Vitamin B5	Blue cheese, brewer's yeast, corn, eggs, lentils, liver, lobster, meats, peanuts, peas, soybeans, sunflower seeds, wheatgerm, wholegrain products
Vitamin B6	Avocados, bananas, bran, brewer's yeast, carrots, filberts, lentils, rice, salmon, shrimps, soybeans, sunflower seeds, tuna, wheatgerm, wholegrain flour
Vitamin C	Blackcurrants, broccoli, Brussels sprouts, cabbage, collard greens, grapefruit, green peppers, guava, lemons, oranges, papaya, potatoes, spinach, strawberries, tomatoes, watercress

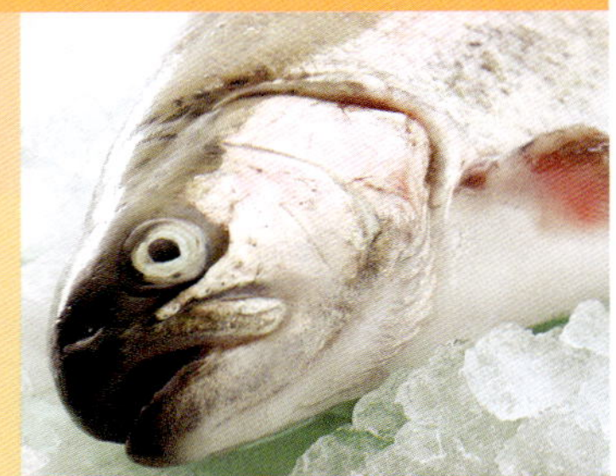

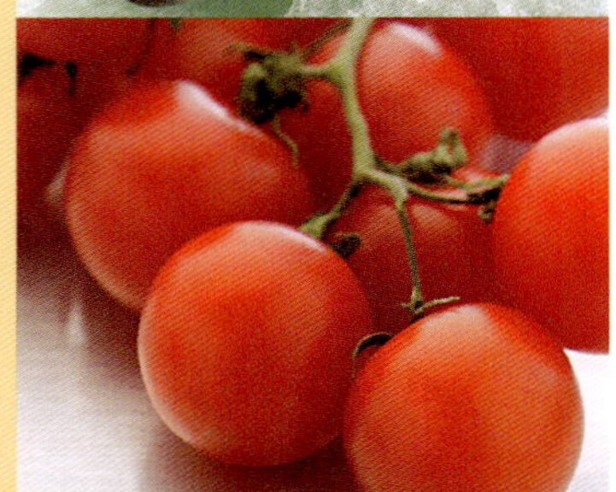

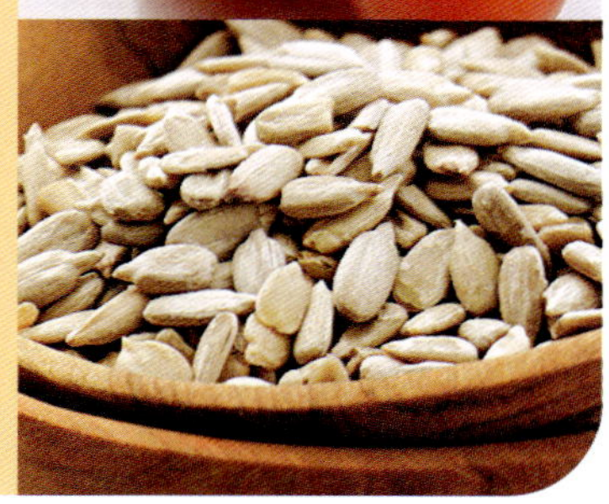

Another stress hormone released by the adrenals is cortisol. Under normal circumstances, cortisol is released on a daily cycle whereby it is higher in the morning, making us feel more alert, and lower at night, helping us to sleep. However, when you have been stressed for some time this rhythm is disrupted. This in turn affects sleep patterns and energy levels and ultimately can make you depressed. Being depressed reduces your body's ability to cope with stress—it is a downward spiral.

Serotonin and dopamine—the mood boosters

Biochemically, mood state is very much dependent on having enough of two particular neurotransmitters (brain-messenger molecules): serotonin and dopamine. When levels of these are low, mood is likely to follow, leaving you ill-equipped to cope with stress. (Many common antidepressant drugs are designed to increase levels of serotonin and dopamine.) With ongoing stress, the over-production of epinephrine and cortisol interfere with the body's careful orchestration of hormones. For example, cortisol appears to interfere with how much serotonin and dopamine is actually produced. Cortisol also reduces the body's sensitivity to these important neurotransmitters.

Supporting your stress response through diet

The aim of the advice given here is to help you to balance your mood by supporting your body's stress response with a diet that puts minimum strain on the adrenal glands. There is no quick fix for regenerating the adrenals and restoring the body's ability to cope with stress. However, one of the first steps is to follow a strategy designed to balance your blood-sugar levels, as summarized on pages 12–17. When blood-sugar levels are low, serotonin and dopamine fall, and so until this mechanism is brought back into an even rhythm, you are unlikely to break the stress cycle. Make sure you include protein-rich foods—such as eggs, fish, lean meat, poultry, dairy products, or soy—in each meal to slow down the rate at which sugar is released into your bloodstream. If necessary, have snacks such as fruit with nuts or yogurt in between meals. Eat small, regular meals throughout the day. This way, you do not let your blood sugar dip.

It is also important that you limit your intake of "stimulants"—such as sugar and sugary foods or drinks, refined foods (including cookies or white bread), coffee, tea, alcohol, and cigarettes—which trigger the body's stress response by provoking a sudden, dramatic rise in blood-sugar levels.

Essential fats (see pages 26–9) are also needed to help break the vicious cycle of an exaggerated stress response. The fats found in foods such as oily fish, nuts, and seeds help improve the health of every cell in your body; by doing this, they ensure that the substances that go in and out of each cell (for example, water, nutrients, hormonal messages, and waste products) are properly regulated. These fats also moderate the body's production of natural inflammatory substances, which in excess encourage the release of too much cortisol.

Nutrients and herbs for adrenal support

In addition to a healthy diet that helps balance blood-sugar levels, there are certain nutrients (see box, opposite) and herbs that particularly nourish overworked adrenals. The key nutrients are vitamins C and B5, alongside vitamins B3 and B6. Herbs that support and regulate the adrenals include licorice, ginseng, and astragalus. Rather than taking each of these substances individually, it is best to find a nutrient-herbal blend that is specifically synergized to have a greater effect than the sum of its parts. Your healthfood-store advisor or healthcare practitioner will be able to help you with this.

Walking and talking

Exercise also plays a part in restoring the health of the adrenals, but not in the way you may expect. Many people who have fast-paced lives that exhaust their adrenals also follow a very rigorous exercise routine, not realizing that this, too, acts as a stressor. When you are run down, doing a hard workout at the gym is the last thing you need. Exercise itself increases levels of epinephrine and cortisol, which is partly why, when you have just finished the work-out, you may feel particularly good. However, if you are suffering from adrenal burn out, this temporary high only exacerbates the problem. If you are experiencing stress symptoms, it is far better to do more moderate exercise—for example, walking, gentle swimming, or yoga—that tones your muscles while only slightly increasing your heart rate.

Finally, no dietary changes will restore your adrenal function to normal if you do not tackle any external sources of stress. This may involve reassessing your work, home, or social life. If the stress is ongoing and you reach the stage where you feel you cannot cope, it is important to seek support. Talk to a sympathetic partner, friend, relative, or co-worker, or enlist the help of a life coach or professional counselor (see pages 134–5).

GOOD-MOOD SUMMARY

To improve your body's stress response:

- eat small meals five or six times a day, and include some fiber- and protein-rich foods in each one
- at least three times a week, eat pumpkin, sunflower, sesame, hemp, and flax seeds and/or oil-rich fish, such as salmon, mackerel, sardines, tuna, or herring
- avoid "stimulants", such as sugar and sugary foods or drinks, refined foods (including cookies or white bread), coffee, tea, alcohol, and cigarettes
- see pages 80–125 for a range of healthy recipe, meal, and snack ideas
- take a blend of nutrients designed to support your adrenal glands (see page 128)
- at least three times a week, take moderate exercise, such as walking, gentle swimming, or yoga
- take steps to reduce stressful issues in your life, ideally calling on someone else who can help

Although the list of symptoms that can result from even a mild nutrient deficiency is seemingly endless, mood swings, irritability, tiredness, and poor concentration are all classic signs that your brain, and the rest of your body, are not receiving all the nutrients they need.

nutrient supplies

Every single process and chemical reaction that takes place in your body depends on a regular supply of "micro" nutrients, such as vitamins and minerals, as well as "macro" nutrients, including protein, carbohydrates, fats, and water, which we need in larger amounts. It makes sense, then, that the raw materials you feed your body affect the way it works, and therefore have an impact on your moods and energy levels.

Nutrients for mood

If we are to avoid mood swings, we need healthy nerves, optimum levels of neurotransmitters (brain messenger molecules, see page 62), and balanced blood-sugar levels (see pages 12–17). Indeed, pretty much all the systems in our body need to be in good working order, even those governing our digestion and detoxification (see pages 30–35). Without a good supply of nutrients, these systems will still work, but they may not function as well as they should. For example, we know that a deficiency in vitamin C causes scurvy, characterized by cracks at the corners of the mouth and mouth ulcers. Although such severe vitamin deficiencies are now rare in developed countries, research has shown that even slightly reduced nutrient levels are clearly linked to a decline in mood.

If you are feeling blue, the chances are that you are not going to have much of an appetite, or if you do, you probably won't crave particularly nutritious foods. So you are likely to find yourself caught up in the vicious circle of feeling low, not eating well, not getting a good supply of nutrients, and feeling lower. People who are depressed, however mildly, are more likely to reach for a bar of chocolate than a bunch of carrots.

Deficiencies in certain nutrients, particularly some of the B vitamins, are clearly associated with depression. In fact, a deficiency in most of the B vitamins is linked to some sort of decline in mental or emotional state: depression, fatigue, confusion, memory loss, apathy, anxiety, irritability, nervousness, sleep disturbances, sluggishness, or loss of appetite. Vitamin B1 (thiamine) was originally known as the "nerve vitamin" because its deficiency causes beri beri, a nerve disease. A severe deficiency of vitamin B3 (niacin) is called pellagra—as well as skin redness and digestive problems, symptoms of pellagra include fatigue, insomnia, apathy, and even manic depression. Folic acid, another member of the B-vitamin family, is believed to be the most commonly deficient nutrient in the world—recent research in the UK found that more than half of girls in their late teens were getting less than the recommended amount of folic acid from their diet. The most common symptom of a folic-acid deficiency is depression.

BITE-SIZE SOLUTION

When you are choosing your food, ask yourself how close to its natural state it is. The more processed or refined a food is, the less likely it is to be rich in the nutrients that nature intended us to have.

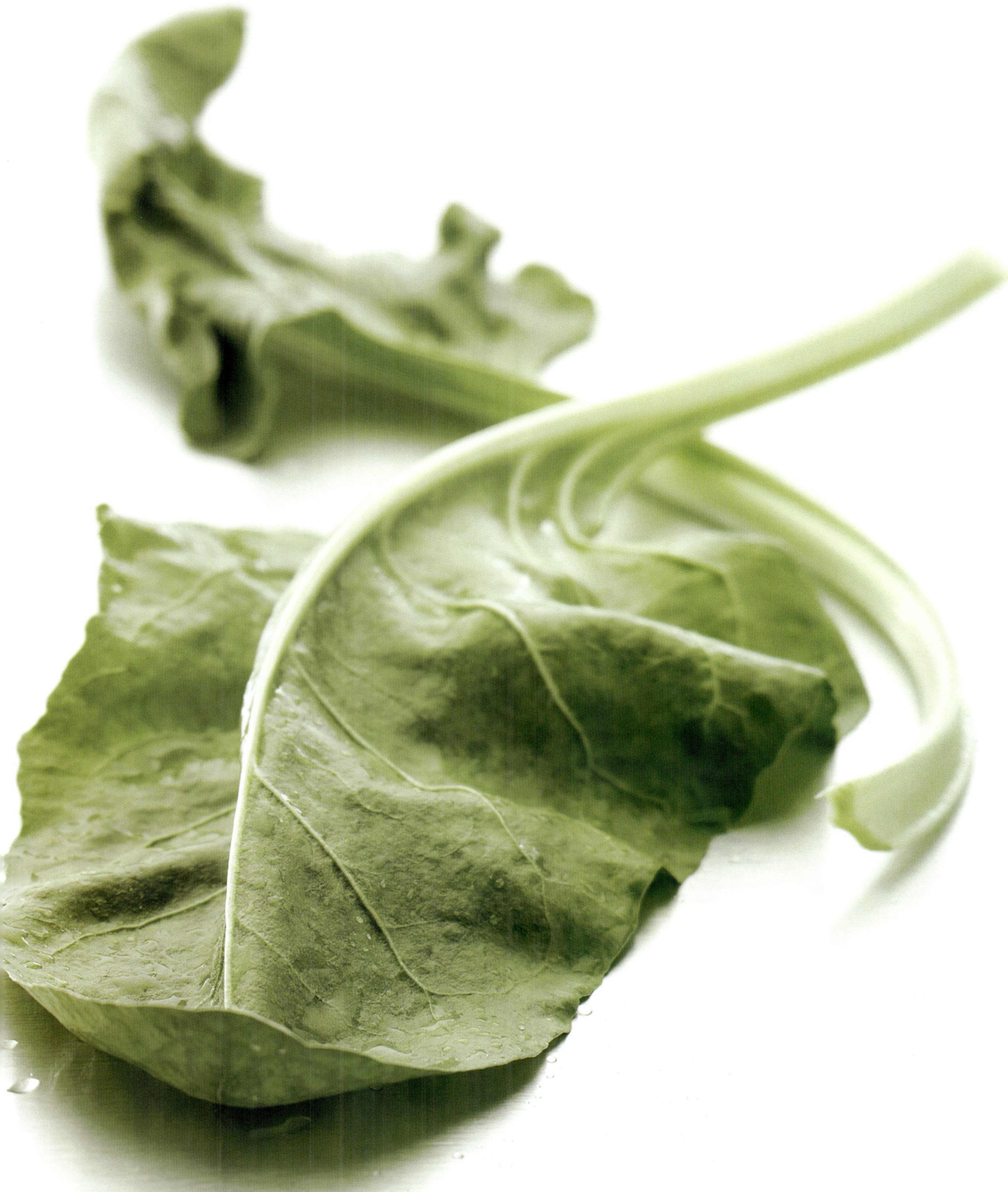

BARE ESSENTIALS FOR FEELING GOOD

For a list of foods that are rich in many of the nutrients mentioned here, see the chart on pages 130–131.

	Role	Nutrients needed
Serotonin	Feel-good neurotransmitter. Needed for good moods, healthy sleep patterns, and appetite control	Vitamins B3, B6, biotin, folic acid, tryptophan, zinc
Dopamine	Stimulating neurotransmitter. Needed for feeling motivation and pleasure	Vitamins B3, B6, B12, C, copper, folic acid, iron, magnesium, manganese, phenylalanine, tyrosine, zinc
Healthy neurons	Nerve cells required for general health and to transmit messages efficiently	Antioxidants, B vitamins, calcium, essential fatty acids, folic acid, magnesium
Even blood-sugar levels	Dives in blood sugar send mood, energy, and concentration crashing	B vitamins, chromium, magnesium, vanadium, zinc

The box above gives an indication of why B vitamins in particular, but also all others, are needed to produce sufficient neurotransmitters, maintain healthy nerves, and keep blood sugar balanced.

The mineral magnesium is vital if nerve cells (neurones) are to communicate effectively with one another. In the absence of sufficient magnesium, the messages passed between nerve cells using neurotransmitters become excessively "loud" and can cause more extreme emotional reactions, including moodiness and agitation.

Essential fatty acids (EFAs) also play a crucial role in nerve messaging. See pages 26–9 for an explanation of how EFAs affect nerve cells and how to include more of the foods that are rich in EFAs in your diet.

How many nutrients are we really getting?

Clearly, a diet that is rich in nutrients can improve your brain function and help you to combat low moods. But how can you ensure that your intake of nutrients is adequate?

One school of thought is that if you have a balanced diet you are getting all the nutrients you need. However, it is important to remember that a great many of us do not actually eat a balanced diet. At worst, we might grab a sugary muffin for breakfast, nibble cookies mid-morning, have a white-bread sandwich with margarine and cheese for lunch, and then eat a convenience meal in the evening. Even if our diet is not that bad, too few of us eat a varied diet of fresh, unprocessed, nutrient-rich foods most of the time.

Most governments have set recommended daily amounts of vitamins that each of us require, based on our sex and age (see page 128). But the truth is that nobody knows exactly how much each of us needs, especially given our individual lifestyles, exercise routines, and environments, let alone our genes. Government recommendations are probably conservative estimates and are generally aimed at the minimum amounts of micro-nutrients required to prevent the symptoms of deficiencies, rather than to optimize health.

Worryingly, research worldwide has shown that significant

numbers of men, women, and children are currently not even getting these minimum recommended daily amounts of nutrients. For example, one survey in the UK found that 72 percent of women and 42 percent of men did not have an adequate intake of magnesium.

As for the macro-nutrients—protein, fats, and carbohydrates—most people in developed countries do get enough of these from their diet. That said, the form in which macro-nutrients are commonly consumed is often not very healthy. We tend to eat refined flour in bread, high-fat animal protein, and excess animal fats or fats that have been processed; many of the micro-nutrients contained in these foods have been lost during processing.

Maximizing your nutrient intake

Leading busy lives and eating on the run mean that many of us are not digesting and absorbing our food well, or even choosing the most nutritious foods in the first place. To ensure that you are getting adequate nutrients from your diet, you need to follow some basic guidelines.

Highly processed and overcooked foods are robbed of their nutrients, yet call on those we do have in our bodies in order to be metabolized. Therefore, it is very important to eat as much fresh, unprocessed, unrefined food as possible. Be careful not to overcook food, as heat destroys many valuable nutrients—try to steam or quickly stir-fry vegetables, for example, and enjoy eating them "crunchy," rather than boiling them until they are completely soft. Whenever possible, eat vegetables raw. The closer a food is to its natural state when you eat it, the more nutrients it will provide. It is also important to eat a variety of foods to ensure that you are getting the full spectrum of required nutrients. Even the healthiest food, if eaten repeatedly, may leave you short of the nutrients it does not contain.

Is a "balanced" diet enough?

Sadly, eating fresh, unprocessed food will not guarantee that your body gets all the nutrients it needs. The balanced-diet argument is partly based on the notion that our soils are rich in minerals that are absorbed by the plants growing in them, which we subsequently eat. Yet with today's intensive farming methods and artificial fertilizers, plants no longer need naturally mineral-rich soil to grow into the bumper-crop, over-sized, uniform fruits and vegetables we now expect to see on our supermarket shelves. Also, we do not always eat fruit and vegetables in season—many have been picked before they are ripe, stored for long periods of time, and shipped across the world, none of which does their nutrient content much good. (In contrast, frozen foods may be richer in nutrients because they are picked at their optimum ripeness and immediately preserved by the freezing process.) Ideally, your balanced diet should consist of as many organic foods as possible, bought fresh from producers who do not use chemicals.

The deficit of nutrients in our food is not the only factor that can leave us low in essential goodness. We are also exposed to many anti-nutrients—substances that deplete our stock of nutrients when they are processed in our bodies. Sodas, sugar, coffee, tea, alcohol, and cigarettes interfere with our body's ability to absorb minerals. By dramatically reducing your consumption of these "anti-nutrients," you can boost your body's intake of vital health- and mood-enhancing nutrients.

If you are worried that you may be lacking in certain nutrients, you should see a qualified nutritionist, who will be able to carry out some deficiency tests and suggest improvements to your diet to overcome any deficiencies.

GOOD-MOOD SUMMARY

To maximize your nutrient levels:

- eat fresh food
- eat a varied diet
- eat foods that have not been highly refined or processed
- limit your intake of "anti-nutrients": alcohol, coffee, tea, sodas, sugar, fried food, highly processed food
- see pages 80–125 for healthy recipe, meal, and snack ideas
- if you are feeling a bit run down or tired, take a multi-vitamin and a vitamin-B complex supplement
- for a full assessment of your nutrient status, visit a nutritionist who will be able to give you guidance on your individual requirements

Many people assume that all fat is bad for them. However, some fats—called essential fatty acids—are not only healthy, but play a vital role in brain function. Increasing your intake of these "good" fats and eating less of the "bad" fats can have a noticeable impact on your moods.

healthy fats

On the list below, tick any of the symptoms that you experience regularly:

- ☐ dry skin
- ☐ acne
- ☐ dermatitis
- ☐ eczema
- ☐ psoriasis
- ☐ allergies
- ☐ fatigue
- ☐ cracked nails
- ☐ dry, limp hair
- ☐ aching joints/arthritis
- ☐ depression
- ☐ high blood pressure

If you suffer from any of the above symptoms, your diet could be lacking in essential fatty acids, or EFAs.

The link between mood problems and a diet that is low in certain essential fats is not new. In *The Anatomy of Melancholy*, published in 1621, the English clergyman and scholar Robert Burton recommended eating a diet low in animal fats but high in borage (otherwise known as starflower) oil and fish. For severe cases of melancholy, he suggested eating cow brains. Although cow brains are hardly considered palatable these days, we now know that they, like borage oil and fish, are rich sources of fatty acids. These fats have been shown to form part of healthy cell membranes and are crucial to the wellbeing of our brain and nervous system.

Good fat, bad fat

Not all fats are the same—some have a very positive impact on wellbeing and we are wise to incorporate them in our daily diet. Broadly known as essential fatty acids, these fats promote good health. They are needed for a healthy heart, brain, nervous system, hormones, skin, water balance, and immunity, to name but a few. However, other fats—the ones we tend to have more of in our diet—are not essential. While it is absolutely fine to eat them in small quantities, high amounts of the less healthy fats—for example, animal fats in meat or milk products, coconut fat, fat absorbed into fried foods, or any fats contained in highly processed foods such as cookies—are actually detrimental to our physical and mental wellbeing.

Every one of our cells is surrounded by a skin of its own, called a membrane, as is each working part within every cell. As you can imagine, the quality of these membranes partly determines the quality of our overall health—after all, on one level, our bodies are simply a mass of cells. One of the main components of cell membranes is fat.

BITE-SIZE SOLUTION

If you're not a great fan of fish, you can get a good intake of omega-3 fats (see page 29) by eating flax and hemp seeds ground up on cereals, soups, or salads. See the High-Five Seeds mix on page 82. Otherwise, make meals that temper the flavor of fish, such as Salmon Rolls (page 106).

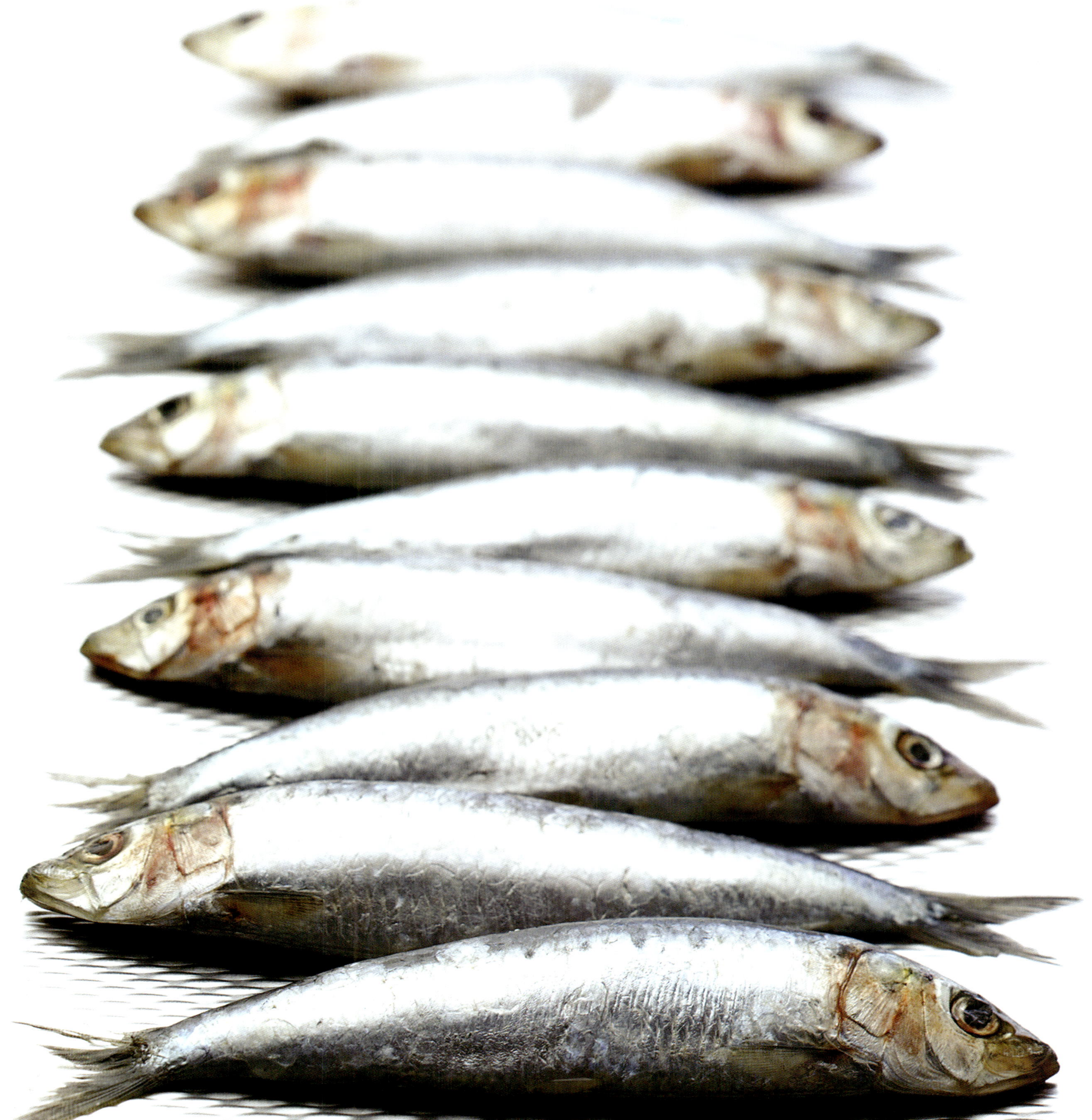

Types of fats

The type of fats that we eat have a considerable impact on our health. There are three main types of dietary fat (also known as lipids): triglycerides, phospholipids, and sterols (such as cholesterol).

Most body fats and almost all the fats we eat are triglycerides, the most common type of fat. Triglycerides can be either saturated or unsaturated, which refers to their chemical structure. Saturated fats—those mainly found in animal products such as meat, butter, and dairy foods, as well as coconut—are more rigid in structure than unsaturated fats and are not actually needed from your diet. Because of this, it is important to limit the amount of saturated fats you eat. Considered to be far more healthy than saturated fats, unsaturated fats are found in vegetable sources, including oils such as olive, sunflower, safflower, rapeseed, soy, peanut, and sesame.

Unsaturated fats can be further subdivided into monounsaturated and poly-unsaturated fats. Olive oil (see box, below) is rich in monounsaturated fat.

Poly-unsaturated fats is another name for essential fatty acids (EFAs), which we already know perform important structural and functional jobs in the body.

EFA families

EFAs are converted in the body (with the help of certain vitamins and minerals) into more concentrated versions of the fats and other substances. These are put to very good use in balancing hormones, keeping skin soft, and more. However, it is the role of the EFAs in ensuring that brain cells and neurotransmitters work efficiently that makes them such an important factor in maintaining stable moods and optimum brain power (see also page 62).

There are two families of EFAs: omega 3 and omega 6. Omega-6 essential fatty acids are found in vegetable oils, such as sunflower and rapeseed oils (both of which are often used in margarines), and also evening-primrose oil and borage (starflower) oil.

In today's typical diet, it is common to have a higher intake of omega-6 fats than omega 3, yet for optimum health and stable moods, a balance of the two is necessary. Combinations of these "good" fats are found in

A WORD ABOUT OLIVE OIL

Any fat or oil should be eaten in moderation, and olive oil, while no exception to this rule, is certainly one of the healthiest fats, especially if it is extra virgin and cold pressed. Olive oil contains seven percent omega-6 fats which, in a cold-pressed olive oil, retain all their healthy properties. The oil is made up of 75 percent mono-unsaturated fat, which means that when used for cooking it is less susceptible to being damaged by heat and turning into a harmful trans-fat (see page 29). For this reason, it is a much better oil to use for cooking than any of the poly-unsaturated ones, such as sunflower oil. What's more, several scientific studies have shown the traditional Mediterranean diet, which is high in olive oil, to protect against many illnesses, including heart disease.

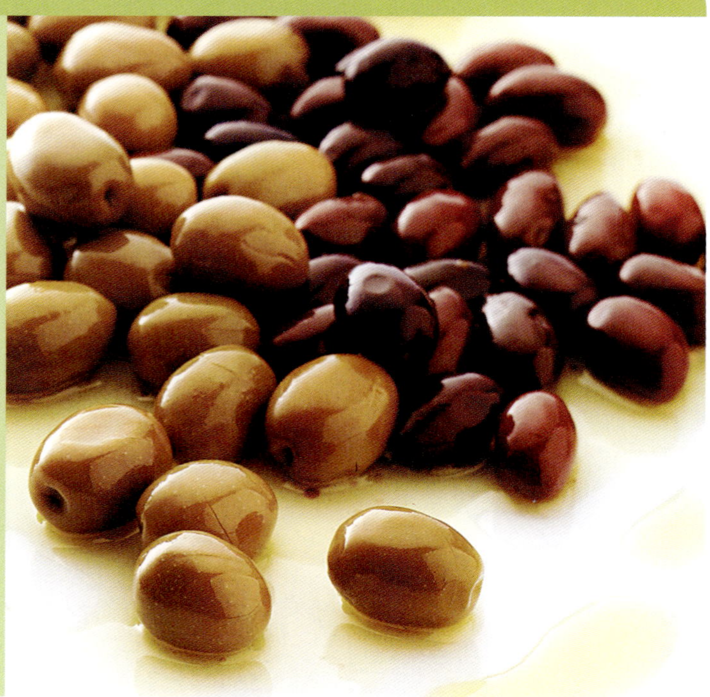

LET YOUR SKIN BE YOUR JUDGE

Your skin can provide a good indication of whether you are giving your whole body enough EFAs. Your body sees skin as less important than your other organs, and so it is last in line for receiving nutrients. Although dry skin can be a symptom of numerous underlying conditions, many people find that by simply taking supplements of flaxseed oil—one tablespoon, or three 1000-mg capsules daily—their skin texture improves considerably. That way, you can also be sure that your other organs, including your brain, are getting ample EFAs.

particularly high amounts in seeds such as sunflower, sesame, pumpkin, hemp, and flax.

Omega-3 fats

Omega-3 essential fatty acids—found in pumpkin and hemp seeds, walnuts, and flaxseed oil, as well as oil-rich fish such as mackerel, herring, pilchards, sardines, salmon, and fresh tuna—are particularly important for emotional and mental health. It is no coincidence that in societies such as those in the Arctic Circle or islands such as Taiwan, where people live on traditional fish-based diets, there are significantly lower incidences of heart disease and depression than in most Western nations. Scientists have actually found that lower consumption of omega-3 fatty acids correlates with increasing rates of depression. Indeed, one report showed that rates of depression in North America and Europe are 10 times higher than in Taiwan. The message is simple: Eat more oily fish! Try to have some at least three times a week.

Trans-fats

The problem with essential fatty acids is that they are very sensitive to damage from a combustion process called oxidation, which can transform "good" fats into what is known as a trans-fatty acid (an unhealthy fatty acid). This slight change has dramatic effects on the way in which the fat can be used in the body and ultimately on our health, including our moods and memory.

If the fats that have already been incorporated into body structures—for example, in cell membranes—are damaged by oxidation, or "hydrogenated," the way those structures work is impaired. To extend their shelf-life, many processed oils and margarines have been heated and treated, forming trans-fats; many convenience foods also contain trans-fats. Try to avoid sources of trans-fats in your diet. If you do eat processed foods, check the labels to make sure they don't mention hydrogenated fat, and store cold-pressed oils and fresh seeds in the refrigerator, where they are protected from rancidity caused by heat, light, and oxygen exposure.

Antioxidant nutrients, such as vitamins A, C, E, selenium, sulfur, and zinc, provide further protection for the essential fats in your body, so it is important to include plenty of antioxidant-rich foods in your diet (see pages 22–5).

GOOD-MOOD SUMMARY

To optimize your body's supply of essential fats:

- have one tablespoon of cold-pressed, unrefined seed oil on salads, stirred into soups, on oatmeal, or neat daily
- grind a blend of pumpkin, sunflower, sesame, hemp, and flax seeds (see page 82) and sprinkle on cereal, soup, and salads daily
- use whole pumpkin, sunflower, and sesame seeds as snacks or sprinkled on cereal or salads
- eat oil-rich fish (such as salmon, mackerel, sardines, tuna, herring, Antarctic ice fish) at least three times a week
- limit your intake of saturated fats from meat, dairy produce, coconut milk
- avoid all refined, processed oils, including processed foods containing them (look out for "hydrogenated fat" in the list of ingredients)
- use olive oil for cooking
- avoid fried foods—broil, bake, poach, or steam instead
- eat plenty of fresh fruit and vegetables to maximize your intake of antioxidants

How you feel is, to a large extent, dictated by how well your body is digesting food, absorbing nutrients, detoxifying, and eliminating waste. Although your brain may seem a long way from your gut, liver, and bowels, it relies on them in order to function effectively.

waste disposal

Tick on the list below any symptoms that you experience regularly:

- ☐ bad breath
- ☐ frequent burning sensation when you urinate
- ☐ fullness in stomach
- ☐ difficulty digesting fatty foods
- ☐ flatulence or bloating or excessive belching
- ☐ diarrhea
- ☐ fewer than one bowel movement a day
- ☐ recurrent headaches
- ☐ sensitivity to chemicals, pollution, cigarette smoke, perfumes
- ☐ spots or acne
- ☐ poor tolerance of alcohol

If you suffer from any of the above, you may well not be digesting or detoxifying properly. The health of your gut—how well you are digesting and absorbing your food—has considerable consequences for the rest of your body. And the workings of your liver—your body's main organ of detoxification—are inextricably bound with your digestive tract. Therefore, your liver and your gut together have an impact on your overall health, including your mood and energy. Your mood, energy, and stress levels also play a significant role in the efficacy of your gut and liver function.

Your body as a food processor

When the food you eat reaches your stomach, a substance called hydrochloric acid there begins the digestive process. The partially digested food then passes into the small intestine, where digestion continues with the help of digestive enzymes that break down the food into small enough particles to be absorbed across the intestinal lining. The remaining "food" then passes into the large intestine, or colon, where some more absorption of nutrients takes place and what is left is prepared for elimination from the body. The nutrients that are absorbed are carried directly to the liver, where they are sorted out, pulled apart, repackaged and sent off for distribution around the body or back to the gut for elimination. Digestion is, theoretically, straightforward and, in an ideal world, this whole process runs smoothly all the time.

However, because of the number of variables to do with our diet, eating habits, and body processes—what we eat, how much we eat, how well we are producing stomach and intestinal juices, how efficiently our guts are moving food along, the acidity of the gut, the balance of bacteria in the intestines, the amount of water present to support the

BITE-SIZE SOLUTION

Your liver is constantly detoxifying all sorts of substances, and the less you burden it on a daily basis, the better the job it will do for you. One way of unburdening your liver is to cut down on alcohol. Aim to have no more than four to six glasses of wine or shots of spirits per week and try to keep some weeks completely alcohol-free.

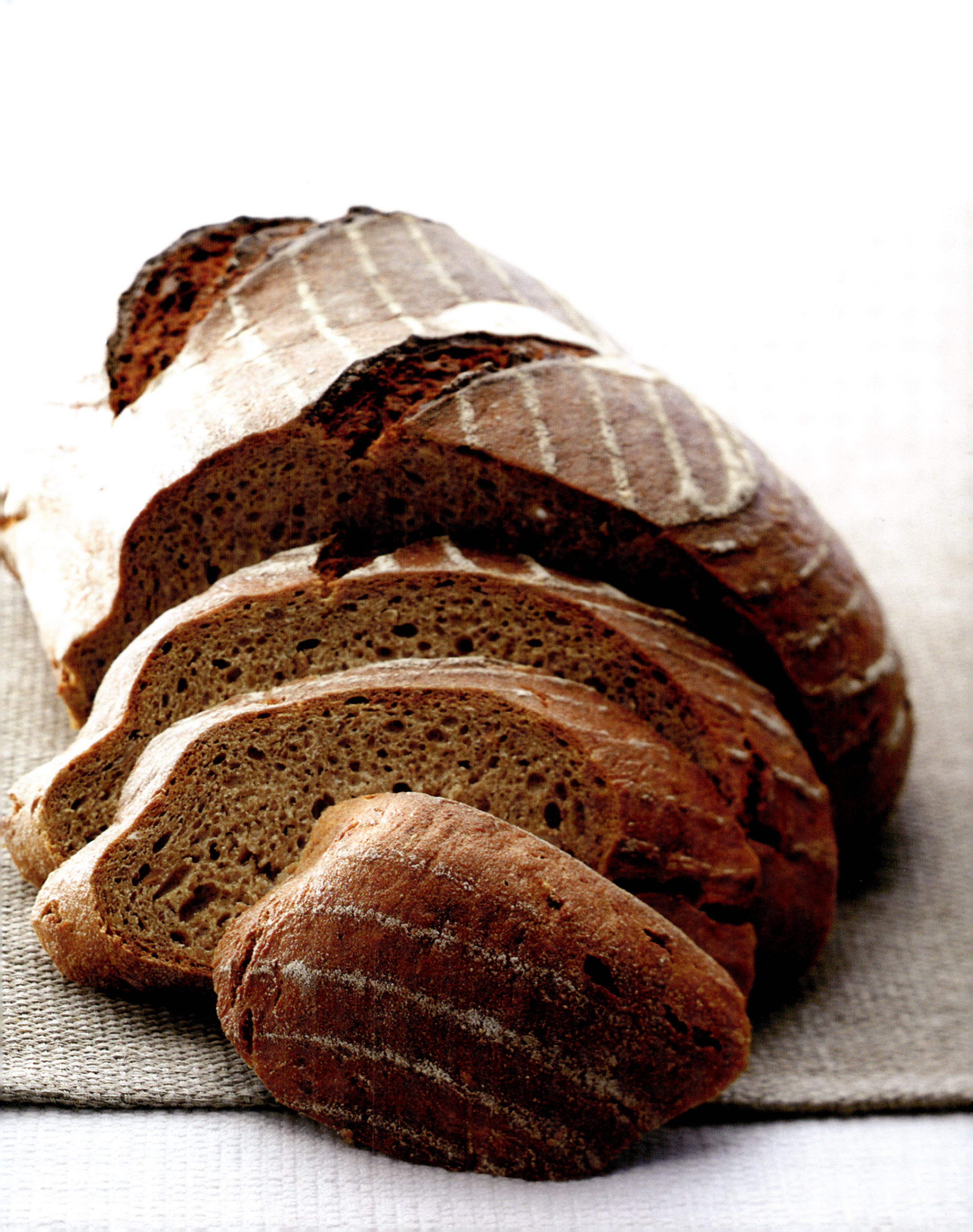

process—there is plenty that can go wrong. If there is even one glitch somewhere in the digestive system, there is much that can be knocked out of balance, even as far away as your brain, affecting how you feel emotionally.

Burdening the system

If your diet consists of foods that are highly refined, high in animal or processed fats, low in fiber, laden with sugar, or generally not as rich in nutrients as they could be, and you are also drinking too much coffee, tea, or alcohol and not enough water, you are stacking up the odds against good digestion and detoxification.

This is all worsened by stress: When you are under pressure, your body diverts most of its energy to dealing with the stress, rather than doing jobs it perceives as unimportant at that moment—one of which is digestion. So when you are stressed, none of the processes in the digestive tract—the production of digestive juices, the movement of food along the gut, the breakdown and absorption of nutrients—is likely to be working efficiently. Yet you are probably still eating food, which ends up not being processed properly. This means you suffer from indigestion, bloating, constipation, or other digestive problems.

Toxic exposure

The liver is the body's main detoxification factory. In addition to the nutrients carried to the liver from the digestive tract, any other substances that happen to get across the gut lining are also taken there. Unfortunately, these substances sometimes include toxins and food particles that have not been completely digested, especially if stress or other problems mean that you are not digesting food correctly. Our normal metabolic processes also produce chemicals within the body that need to be detoxified and eliminated.

We are all constantly exposed to countless external toxins. Our environments are increasingly filled with substances that our bodies have to process in order to render them harmless. Toxins processed in the liver are passed through into the gut to be carried out of the body. If you are not eliminating waste via your bowels properly or

TOXIC METALS

A number of problems involving low mood, fatigue, and poor mental function have been traced to particularly high levels of certain toxic metals in the body. For example, we are all exposed to small amounts of lead, in the air we breathe. Other metals, such as mercury (from amalgam fillings and contaminated fish), aluminium (from pans, foil, and certain medications), and cadmium (from cigarette smoke), can also accumulate in the body.

Although most of us can cope with small amounts of such metals, in higher amounts or in particularly sensitive people they can have a detrimental effect on the nervous system (including the brain) and other parts of the body. Some dentists have found that patients with symptoms such as fatigue and mood problems, as well as panic attacks, irritability, poor memory, confusion, and many other symptoms, recover when their amalgam fillings are replaced with ceramic ones. This must be done by an experienced dentist to avoid even more mercury escaping into the body when the old fillings are drilled out.

If you suspect that you may have been exposed to high levels of these metals, you can have a hair-mineral analysis done by a healthcare practitioner. This involves taking a small sample of hair, which is tested for levels of toxic and other metals in the body's tissues. Based on the results, you can then find ways to minimize your exposure to the offending substance and go on a special detoxification program designed to chelate, or "claw out," the toxic metals. For example, pectin (found in apples) and alginic acid (found in seaweed) are able to bind to certain metals and escort them out of the body. Ensuring that you are getting adequate levels of zinc and calcium, which act as antagonists to lead, can reduce an accumulation of this harmful metal in the body.

regularly, the toxins are more likely to hang around and be circulated in the body.

Poor digestion and mood

You only have to remember how low you felt on a Sunday, having consumed a large amount of alcohol the previous Friday night, to see what a dampening effect overloading your liver can have on your mood and energy. Or, if you are not much of a drinker, you may notice how overeating fatty, processed foods for a couple of days leaves you sluggish, lethargic, and unmotivated.

Remember, it is not just how toxic a substance is that makes it harmful, but also how efficiently your body is able to process it. In a sensitive person, any number of substances—those that build up in the body and those that come from the outside—can act as "toxins" and interfere with the body processes that are needed to maintain balanced moods. Basically, what seems to happen is that the build-up of harmful substances owing to poor detoxification interferes with the chemistry of the brain. The mechanisms that control the balance of neurotransmitters such as serotonin—how they are produced and then how efficiently they are transmitted—are so finely tuned that any slight interference caused by toxic overload is likely to disturb these processes.

Also, if the liver is overloaded you end up with an excess of oxidants in the body. Oxidants are harmful molecules that damage cell membranes, which need to be healthy for the transmission of messages in the brain. Given that your mood is in part dictated by the transmission of messages using substances such as serotonin, an inefficient messaging system could well mean that your moods are not as good as they could be.

Help your body to detox

In recent years, as "detox" diets and programs have become fashionable, it has been easy to forget that the body does not detoxify only when we "go on a detox"—it does so permanently. So we would do well to give it a hand constantly, not just for three days every so often after a month of indulgence! Even if we are not particularly excessive, our usual diet, the water we drink, and our environment increasingly place a burden on our detoxification systems.

Managing your diet can be a crucial and relatively easy way to make sure that you are not overburdening your body. By choosing foods and drinks that aid the digestive system rather than overloading it, you can directly reduce the demands on your liver.

Optimizing waste disposal

Given the way in which an overloaded digestive system can overwork the liver, and the impact that this can have on your mood and energy production, it is important to start with a diet that nourishes the gut. This means eating fresh, minimally processed foods that are low in sugar, low in animal and processed fats, high in fiber (see below), and rich in nutrients; it also means keeping "irritants," such as coffee, tea, alcohol, processed foods, and unnecessary additives, to a minimum. By eating like this most of the time (although occasional indulgences are likely to be very good for your mood), you are nourishing yourself and minimizing the load on your system.

The other thing to remember about your food is to take time to relax and enjoy it. By sitting down, chewing well to set up the sequence of processes in your digestive tract, and resting for at least 10 minutes after you have finished eating, you can vastly improve your digestion.

Fiber and antioxidants for detoxification

One of the most important ways of supporting the liver is including plenty of fiber in your diet. Fiber is not just about having your morning prunes to stave off constipation. Having regular bowel movements is almost as important for your health as putting good food in your mouth, because it means that you are eliminating waste products effectively. Fiber not only keeps your gut moving, it also binds onto toxins in the gut and escorts them out of the body. The chart on page 34 gives a list of fiber-rich foods.

Another very important group of nutrients for supporting liver detoxification is antioxidants. As their name suggests, they protect us from harmful oxidants. The body has its

NUTRIENTS FOR DIGESTION AND DETOXIFICATION

For good digestion and detoxification, we need a full range of nutrients, which is best obtained from a varied, balanced diet. The following nutrients are particularly important:

Nutrient benefit	Rich food sources
Fiber	Barley, beans (such as black-eyed, garbanzo, kidney, pinto), brown rice, buckwheat, fresh fruit, fresh vegetables, lentils, oats, rye, wholewheat
Antioxidants	Avocado, beets, berries, broccoli, cabbage, carrots, collard greens, fish, garlic, grapes, green tea, nuts, onions, peppers, prunes, raisins, seeds, sweet potatoes, tomatoes, watercress, wheatgerm
Digestive enzymes	Papaya, pineapple
To promote "friendly" bacteria	Asparagus, garlic, Jerusalem artichokes, live natural yogurt, miso, onions

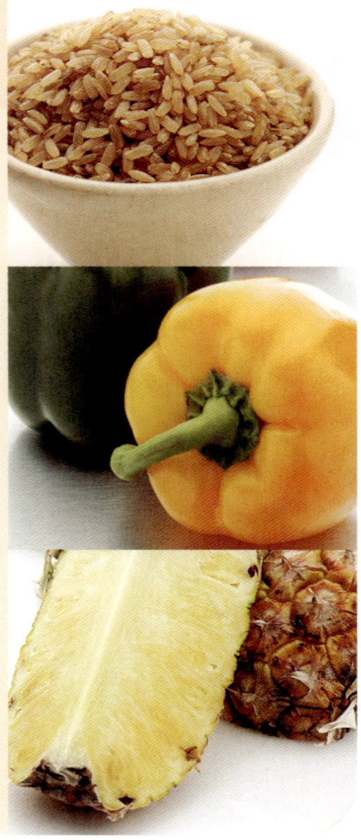

own sophisticated mechanisms for "mopping up" oxidants, but we need to provide a good supply of nutrients to keep them well in check. Antioxidant-rich nutrients include: vitamin A, vitamin C, vitamin E, zinc, selenium, anthocyanidins, glutathione, lycopene, and lipoic acid. The chart above and the nutrient chart on pages 130–131 give lists of foods that are rich in these nutrients. It is worth noting that the colors that are present in fresh fruit and vegetables largely come from the variety of antioxidants they contain. Therefore, it is a good idea to include a wide range of colorful fruit and vegetables in your diet.

Friendly bugs

An important factor in the health of the intestines—and thus a healthier liver and better elimination—is the balance of the right bacteria. We all have billions of them in our gut, but if there is a lack of so-called "friendly" bacteria—a problem often triggered by a diet that is high in sugar and refined foods—"unfriendly" organisms can proliferate. The friendly bacteria are sometimes known as "probiotics" and are found in good quality "live" yogurts, as well as in some dietary supplements. Many of the yeasts, parasites, or

BITE-SIZE SOLUTION

Eating foods that are rich in fiber helps keep your digestion and detoxification systems working well. High-fiber foods are whole grains—such as brown rice, oats, rye, barley, wholewheat, and buckwheat—fresh vegetables, fresh fruit, beans (such as black-eyed, garbanzo, kidney, pinto), and lentils. Designer Muesli (page 83), Mongettes Charentaises (page 91), and Grated Apple Ice (page 121) are all fiber-rich recipes.

TOXINS

Toxins are internal and external substances that place a burden on the body's reserves. The work they represent for the liver depends not just on their inherent toxic properties but also on the body's ability to detoxify them.

What places a burden on the liver?

- alcohol
- prescription drugs—oral contraceptives, high-dose aspirin/acetaminophen, and so on
- recreational drugs
- exposure to chemicals—pesticides, industrial chemicals, paints, solvents, fuels
- a low-fiber, highly refined diet
- excessive fat, protein, calories
- bowel toxicity owing to poor detoxification and elimination
- dietary sources of oxidants—rancid oils, fried or charred foods
- stress

harmful bacteria that can proliferate in an unhealthy gut may cause low-lying digestive symptoms such as bloating (if not more serious problems), and they can also subtly release toxins that affect mood. When a person in such a situation works with a professional healthcare practitioner to eliminate the unwanted organisms and re-establish the levels of friendly bacteria, the improvement in mood and other symptoms can be remarkable.

The best way to "recolonize" your gut with these bacteria is to take a probiotic supplement under the guidance of your nutritionist or healthcare practitioner. If you do not have any digestive or detoxification problems and merely want to keep up your levels of friendly bacteria, eating natural yogurt that is made with live cultures every day can give you a regular supply. Bear in mind that yogurts or yogurt drinks with added sugar usually cancel out any benefit, as sugar tends to feed the "bad" bacteria.

Water for life

All cells contain and are surrounded by water—we need it for life. Many people with constipation find relief just by increasing their water intake. One of the large intestine's jobs is to draw water from the food that arrives there, in order to form feces. If you do not drink enough water, your bowel will draw on as much as it can from the food, leaving a dry, compacted stool—that is, constipation. It is best to drink mineral or filtered water. Only pure water or herbal or fruit teas really count toward your daily intake; coffee, regular tea, juices or cordials, and sodas do not. Aim to drink at least 3 pints (1½ litres) of water throughout the day.

GOOD-MOOD SUMMARY

To optimize your digestion and detoxification:

- have fresh, colorful vegetables raw, lightly steamed, or stir-fried twice a day
- have at least two pieces of fresh fruit daily
- eat plenty of fiber-rich foods, for example beans, lentils, whole grains, fruit, and vegetables
- limit your intake of sugar added to foods and drinks and also foods and drinks that are already sweet, such as candy, chocolate, cookies, cakes, sodas, sweetened juices, etc.
- avoid refined carbohydrates, such as sugar, white bread, pasta, cakes, and so on
- avoid processed, refined, pre-packaged foods, and fast food
- avoid fried and fatty foods—broil, bake, poach, or steam your food instead
- drink at least 3 pints (1½ litres) of pure water throughout the day
- limit your intake of tea and coffee. Good alternatives are various herb/spice/fruit teas, or "coffee substitutes"
- limit your intake of alcohol—ideally no more than 2 to 3 glasses, 2 to 3 times a week
- take time to eat and chew well
- don't eat more than you need to
- see pages 80–125 for healthy recipe, meal, and snack ideas

A 21-DAY CLEANSE

Although, ideally, you should minimize the load on your gut and liver through the kind of diet described on pages 30–35, it can be helpful occasionally to give your body a rest from its daily task of cleansing. Short of doing a full, fasting, detoxification program, there are plenty of steps that you can take to cleanse your body. To lessen the burden, you can boost your body's health with fresh, rejuvenating foods and give it a break from having to deal with foods that overload its normal cleansing routine.

This 21-day program is designed to:

- fuel the body optimally
- kick-start the breaking of bad habits
- cleanse all your body systems
- enhance all your body systems
- restore control and balance to your body and moods

After following such a program, most people find they feel physically energized, and mentally and emotionally reinvigorated. However, if you are ill or on medication, you should not embark on this program without first asking your doctor or nutritionist for advice.

The week before

Gradually start reducing your intake of tea, coffee, alcohol, and sugar, so that you do not have to go "cold turkey" on day one. For some people, such changes are very different to their normal routine, so you may want to introduce them slowly over a couple of weeks before launching fully into the cleansing program. This way, you are being more gentle on your system and you will be less likely to feel unwell as you detox. Make sure you stock up on all the foodstuffs you will need for the program.

Embarking on the program

Once you begin the 21-day program, your daily food intake (organic as far as possible) should include:

- at least 3 pints (1½ litres) of pure water—although this may take some getting used to, it is quite easy to achieve if you start the day with hot water with a squeeze of lemon or grated gingerroot, then have an herbal tea between meals, and a glass of mineral or filtered water before each meal
- three pieces of fresh fruit—vary the fruit you have, and choose those that are in season and, ideally, locally grown, as these are likely to be fresher
- fresh vegetables at lunch and dinner—have a variety and choose different colors
- fresh vegetable and fruit juices—for a particularly cleansing juice add some greens, such as spinach, broccoli, or collard greens, and some fresh ginger. Carrot, apple, celery, grapefruit, collard greens, and ginger juice is particularly delicious.
- plenty of naturally fiber-rich foods, such as beans, lentils, whole grains, and root vegetables (beans are best bought dried, soaked, and then cooked, but you can also buy them canned for convenience)
- for protein, have soy products (such as tofu and tempeh), beans, lentils, sprouted beans, an occasional organic egg or piece of fish. You can buy sprouted beans at healthfood stores or sprout your own.
- for starchy foods, have brown rice, baked potatoes, corn or vegetable pasta, rice noodles, quinoa, buckwheat, rice cakes

It is important to cut out all the things that clog up your digestive system, such as:

- alcohol—to be avoided at all costs
- coffee, tea—have herbal, fruit, and spice teas instead
- meat and poultry
- fried or fatty foods, including fries, potato chips, bacon
- dairy products—for example, cheese, yogurt, cream, buttter, ice cream, fromage frais—with the exception of organic, live, natural yogurt. Use tahini (sesame spread) instead of butter; use soy, almond, or rice milk and soy yogurt.
- any foods containing artificial additives or sweeteners
- processed and refined foods, including "convenience meals"
- sugary foods and drinks—have an occasional fruit bar or sesame snap, or a little fruit or dried fruit instead
- wheat—bread, pasta, crackers, cookies, muffins, wheat

cereals, cous cous, ordinary noodles (including egg noodles), cakes, bagels. Many people who have a food sensitivity (see pages 38–9) find they feel less bloated and lethargic when they cut down on wheat, especially bread.
- limit your intake of other gluten grains—that is oats, rye, and barley—to once every two days

Don't go hungry

While you are following this cleansing program you should never be hungry or skip meals. You will be eating substantial meals consisting of foods that are satisfying because they are so rich in fiber—these foods will provide your body with all the nutrients it needs. If you do feel hungry, don't hesitate to have a snack, such as:

- rice cakes (or oat cakes) with houmous or tahini
- raw vegetables, such as broccoli, cauliflower, sugar-snap peas, red peppers, carrots, celery, baby corn, radishes—dipped in houmous if you like
- half an avocado and a few cherry tomatoes
- fresh fruit
- a small handful of dried fruit (too much may make you bloated)—buy the unsulfured types
- a small handful of almonds, Brazils, cashews, pecans, or walnuts, or pumpkin or sunflower seeds—have only unsalted, unroasted nuts and seeds

To support your diet, also:

- Put 1 tablespoon of organic, golden flaxseeds (available in most healthfood stores, avoid the brown variety) in a glass of water overnight then chew and drink the mixture in the morning. Flaxseeds are cleansing and also help bulk out your food as it passes through the digestive tract.
- Take a liver "flush" first thing each morning: Mix the juice of 1 grapefruit and 1 lemon, 2 tablespoons of extra-virgin olive oil, 1 crushed garlic clove, and a 1-inch (2½-cm) piece of gingerroot (grated).
- Buy a firm-bristle brush from a healthfood store or drug store and brush your skin daily before you shower. This enhances lymphatic flow, which improves waste-disposal mechanisms. Brush in steady upward movements toward the heart.
- Take some exercise daily or at least every other day. This can be walking, swimming, cycling, yoga, or whatever form of exercise you prefer. It is best to avoid particularly vigorous kinds of exercise as they can be too much for the detoxing body.
- Make sure you are getting adequate sleep (at least seven hours a night) so that your body has time to rest and regenerate.

Daily supplements for good digestion and detoxification

You can buy these at healthfood stores, or ask your nutritionist or herbalist to recommend good brands.

- an antioxidant blend that includes vitamin C, vitamin E, beta carotene, selenium, glutathione, lipoic acid, n-acetyl cysteine; good liver function depends on an adequate supply of antioxidant nutrients
- aloe vera juice—various brands do blends that contain herbs to promote cleansing; aloe vera is very soothing, cleansing, and toning for the digestive tract
- milk thistle (100 mg three times daily, standardized to contain 70 percent silymarin), which is particularly supportive for your liver; you may prefer to look for a liver-support blend at your healthfood store that includes other herbs such as dandelion
- digestive enzymes (available in capsule form) to optimize your break down of food

Meal planning

Using recipes from Chapter 3 (pages 80–125), a couple of days' meals may look like this:

BREAKFAST: Apple Oatmeal (page 82) or Very Berry Breaky using soy milk (page 83)
LUNCH: Baked potato with Houmous, Avocado, and Alfalfa topping (page 86) or Spicy Bean Salad (page 89) or Dahl (page 90)
DINNER: Kebabs (page 102) with Spiced Bean Stew (page 113) or Crunchy Carrot Salad (page 116) or Roasted Sweet Vegetables (page 117)

The notion that food sensitivities can affect mood is still seen as controversial by some medical professionals. Yet clinical experience clearly shows that when some people eliminate certain foods from their diet, quite simply, they feel healthier and happier.

food sensitivity

Tick on the list below any symptoms that you experience regularly:

- ☐ lethargy or apathy, particularly after eating
- ☐ feeling better if you don't eat
- ☐ unexplained grogginess/fatigue
- ☐ poor concentration
- ☐ mood swings
- ☐ unexplained aching
- ☐ dark circles under your eyes
- ☐ fluid retention (symptoms of which include a puffy face, swollen ankles, and daily weight fluctuations)
- ☐ food cravings, such as for bread or cheese
- ☐ irritable bowel syndrome/constipation/mild diarrhea

If you suffer from any of the above, you could be sensitive to foods you are eating or substances in your environment.

Defining a food sensitivity

Food sensitivity, or intolerance, is a broad term that describes all unpleasant reactions to food. If you eat a food that you are sensitive to, you may suffer from mild diarrhea, tiredness, or constipation, or you may just feel generally unwell. Not all such reactions occur immediately after eating the food—some scientists suggest that it is a build-up of negative reactions in the body over time that creates symptoms. For example, if you eat bread every day and you are sensitive to it, you may feel groggy and down, but because the symptoms do not come on as soon as you have eaten some bread, you may not make the connection.

A food allergy, on the other hand, is a form of intolerance in which a particular food triggers an abnormal, measurable immune response in the body. Food allergies can cause a range of unpleasant symptoms, such as migraine, asthma, abdominal pain, vomiting, and skin rashes. Allergic symptoms—unlike many reactions caused by a food sensitivity—often appear soon after the food is eaten.

How food sensitivities affect you

The exact mechanism by which a reaction to a food has a detrimental effect on mood is still the subject of conjecture. One theory is that it is often the foods we eat the most that gradually wear out the digestive processes for that particular food, leaving larger particles of foods than is ideal circulating in the body. These particles trigger an inflammatory reaction, which affects, among other things, the brain, nerves, and the neurotransmitters (messenger molecules), such as serotonin,

BITE-SIZE SOLUTION

Wheat is the most common allergen. If you decide to experiment with avoiding wheat, the following are good alternatives that can instead provide the starchy part of your meal: rye bread (make sure it is pure rye flour); other flour breads, such as rice/soy; rice cakes; oat cakes; rye crackers; oatmeal; oat and other grain breakfast cereals; corn/rice/vegetable pasta; rice noodles; brown rice; quinoa; corn; potato; sweet potato; polenta; millet.

COMMON ALLERGY TRIGGERS

- **Wheat:** in bread, cakes, cookies, cereals, muffins, bagels, pasta, pizza
- **Gluten:** in wheat, oats, rye, barley
- **Dairy products:** milk, cheese, ice cream, yogurt, anything else made with milk
- **Mold/yeast:** found on/in nuts, cheeses, dried fruit, mushrooms, sourdough, beer, and so on
- **Corn and corn products** (such as corn oil, starch)
- **Food additives and preservatives:** notably MSG (monosodium glutamate, added to many processed foods and, most notoriously, much Chinese food)
- **Eggs**
- **Chocolate**

which are responsible for our moods. In other words, these inflammatory substances interfere with brain chemistry.

Ironically, we often crave the foods that are doing us the most harm. In another disputed mechanism, the body seems to develop an addiction-like relationship with the foods that are creating symptoms of fatigue and mood swings. Some scientists believe that the proteins in certain foods, most commonly wheat and dairy products, act like natural opiates—giving some relief, temporarily. Yet the come-down after eating these foods is unpleasant, and leaves us craving more. Food sensitivities can also trigger a reaction similar to that caused by plummeting blood-sugar levels—sinking energy, mood, concentration, and a raised heart beat.

Avoidance testing for food sensitivities

The best method of testing for food sensitivities depends on what you suspect you are sensitive to. Blood tests and skinprick tests are available through healthcare practitioners. However, to check for delayed food sensitivities, you can use a method known as avoidance testing at home. Begin by eliminating the foods you suspect you may be sensitive to from your diet. You could try eliminating some of the common allergens listed in the box left, or choose foods that you crave, as these are often allergens. It is best to eliminate one food at a time. After four weeks, reintroduce the eliminated foods (one by one if you've given up more than one, at five-day intervals), by eating a substantial amount of the food (for example, three slices of bread if you have been avoiding wheat) while "pulse testing" your reaction. To do this, take your pulse at rest (sitting or lying down quietly) 10, 30, and 60 minutes before and after you have eaten the food. Compare the speed of your pulse for each time interval before and after eating the food. Note what you started eating and whether you had any reactions, which may vary from an increased pulse within minutes to more prolonged effects, such as feeling groggy for days.

If a food triggers a reaction, avoid it for at least a further six months, after which time you can retest by eating it again. It is best not to reintroduce in large amounts any food you know you are sensitive to. Instead, eat it only occasionally, or certainly not more than once every four days. While avoidance testing, you should ideally work with a healthcare professional to ensure you are not restricting your diet too much, and to improve your digestive and immune systems in order to minimize your body's oversensitivity.

Bear in mind that the challenge with detecting sensitivities is that it may not be a particular food, but a "hidden" ingredient that you are sensitive to, such as mold on nuts, or food additives, or chemicals in water.

GOOD-MOOD SUMMARY

To detect and address any food sensitivities you may have:

- assess which foods you eat daily and which you crave
- eliminate these from your diet, choosing good alternatives (ideally with the help of a healthcare practitioner) to ensure you are not missing out on important nutrients
- follow the guidelines for "pulse testing" with the foods you have eliminated
- limit or avoid foods you appear to be sensitive to, again, making sure your diet is not too restrictive, depriving you of adequate nutrients

MOOD DISORDERS ARE NOW AFFECTING MORE OF US THAN EVER BEFORE. BY GETTING TO GRIPS WITH THE NUTRITIONAL FACTORS THAT LIE AT THE ROOT OF OUR LOW MOODS, WE ARE ABLE TO SEE PRACTICAL, REALISTIC, AND SUSTAINABLE ANTI-DOTES TO CONDITIONS THAT INTERFERE WITH OUR QUALITY OF LIFE.

Conditions that affect your mood, mind, and energy come in many forms and even more degrees of seriousness. You may feel persistently low; you may find that you are often irritable or turning to food for a boost; you may suffer from premenstrual syndrome or seasonal affective disorder; you may have difficulty sleeping or find your brain power is not what it used to be. One thing all these problems have in common is that they are inextricably linked to your diet. In the following pages, we examine in detail a number of mood-related conditions, such as fatigue and binge-eating disorder, and explore how to overcome them using nutritional methods.

mood's many guises

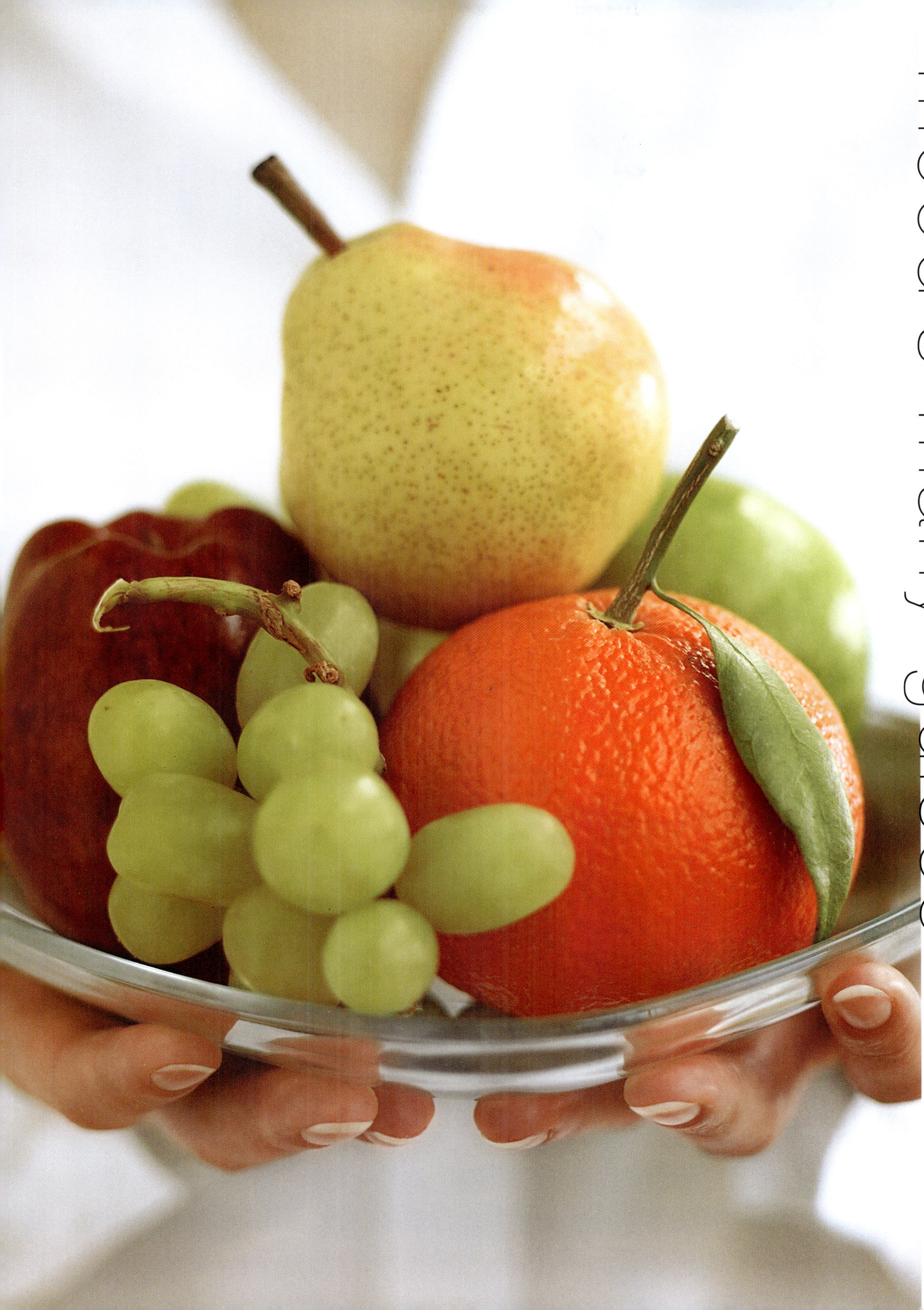

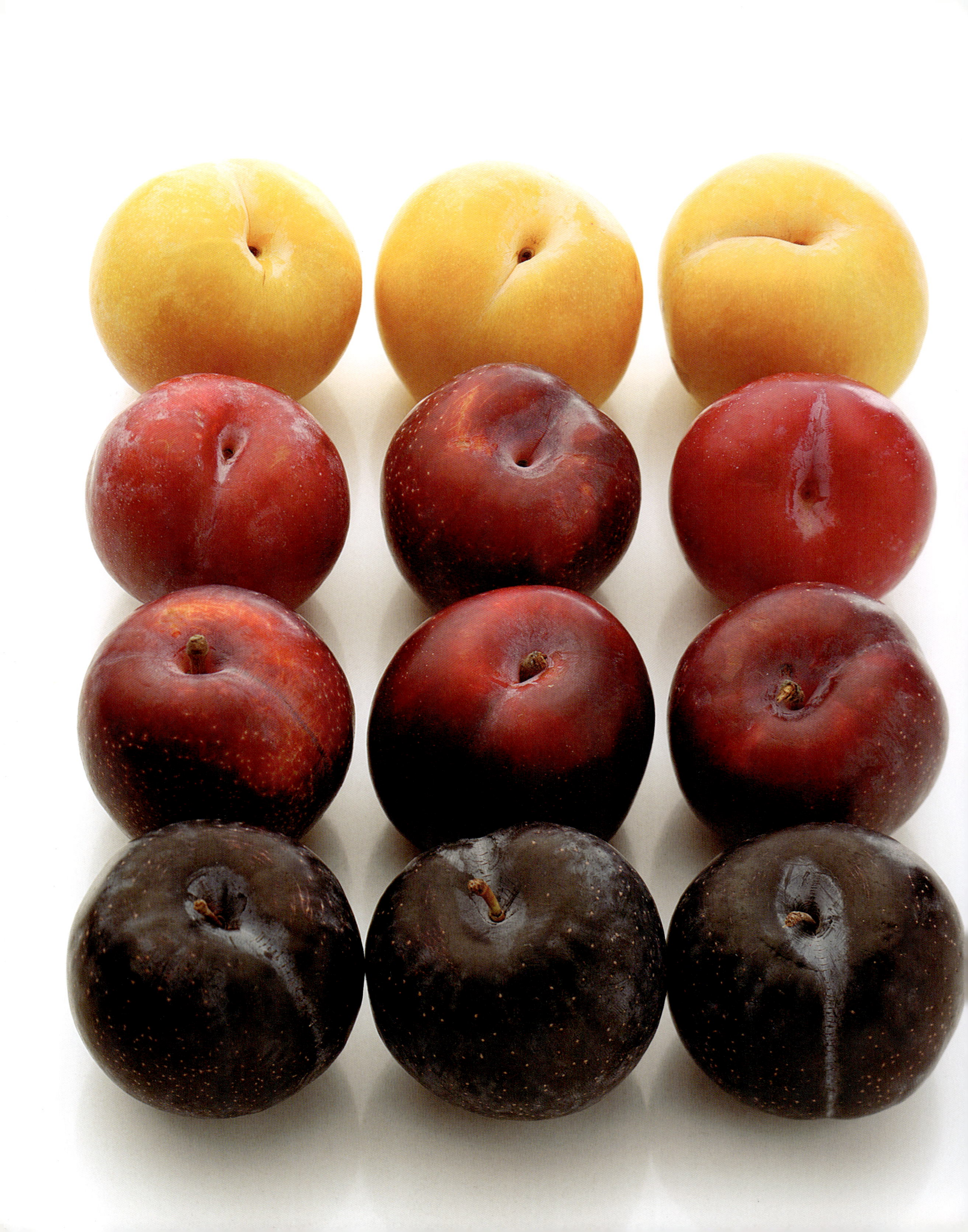

how to use this chapter

Problems with mood, memory, and energy can be low-lying conditions that quietly and subtly undermine our quality of life. They can also be serious: Low moods or lapsing mental sharpness can, of course, take on grave forms such as major depression or Alzheimer's disease. The information in this chapter is aimed at supporting you if you fall into the first category. As a nutritionist, I have described ways of dealing with mild mood disorders through diet. While much of the information in the following chapters could be beneficial across the spectrum of each condition, the suggestions made here are not intended to combat extreme states of illnesses.

The check-lists at the beginning of each section are designed to give you a general indication of the most common symptoms of the milder forms of each problem. Remember, some symptoms can be signs of an underlying disease. It is always advisable to check with your doctor before embarking on any health program, especially if it involves significant changes to your usual diet. Similarly, if you are on medication do check with your physician about making radical changes to your diet or taking any nutritional supplements.

Having said this, adhering to the basic principles of healthy eating can make even the healthiest of people feel even better. It follows that if you provide your body with good quality "fuel", and minimize your intake of substances that silt up your system, both your body and mind will work more efficiently for you. Much research has shown that diet and food supplements can relieve or even eliminate symptoms of all kinds of illnesses, not least those affecting the way our minds work.

The previous chapter outlined the underlying principles of good nutrition, particularly in relation to mood. This chapter is designed to bring together the dietary guidelines that are particularly helpful in treating each mood disorder. You could simply read the section on the condition that interests you. However, for more detail, refer back to sections in Chapter 1, The Physiology of Melancholy, or forward to Chapter 3, Feel Good Food, for advice on how to put those nutritional principles into practice.

Without a good intake of the nutrients needed to produce energy you are likely to end up feeling constantly exhausted, on edge, and irritable. By consuming fresh, unprocessed food and drinks, and avoiding substances that drain your energy, you really can banish perpetual tiredness.

energy deficit

On the list below, tick the symptoms that are familiar and persistent for you:

- ☐ feeling tired all the time
- ☐ using coffee, tea, or a cigarette to get you going in the morning
- ☐ feeling unrefreshed after sleep
- ☐ experiencing energy slumps during the day
- ☐ having mood and concentration swings
- ☐ craving sweet and starchy food, coffee, tea, alcohol, cigarettes
- ☐ getting angry easily
- ☐ over-reacting to pressing or antagonistic issues
- ☐ regularly feeling impatient
- ☐ feeling anxious or nervous

If you ticked five or more symptoms, you will almost certainly feel more energetic if you follow the advice in this section.

Sometimes everything just seems like such an effort, and all you can think of is bedtime. We all have our off days when we feel low in energy, but for many people, this is pretty much a permanent way of life. Yes, it is normal to feel tired after a week of getting up early, working hard, exercising, and going to bed late. But the tiredness some people experience every day is more like a constant, wiped-out, drained feeling. And when you feel that way, it's almost impossible for you not to get tetchy with your family, friends, and coworkers.

Unless you have an underlying illness, your weariness and irritability are probably easily surmountable. With a little effort, you can identify and tackle the root causes of your tiredness and adopt a diet and lifestyle that truly energize you. However, if your tiredness is extreme or prolonged, you should talk to your doctor in order to rule out any potentially serious causes.

Identifying the cause of your tiredness

There is a host of reasons why you may be feeling weary, many of which are simple to overcome. For example, being dehydrated can make you tired. Try drinking at least six glasses of bottled or filtered water daily and you may well quickly see an improvement in your energy levels. Similarly, if you are not eating nutritious foods, you may be missing out on some of the important energy nutrients listed on the chart opposite (see pages 22–5 for more on nutrient deficiencies). Your doctor may find that low iron stores (especially common in women and vegetarians) are at the

BITE-SIZE SOLUTION

To get each day off to a good start, boost your energy levels by having some protein- and carbohydrate-rich foods at breakfast. This prevents your blood sugar—and your energy and mood—plummeting mid-morning, leaving you reaching for a pick-me-up, such as coffee or a doughnut. Try some of the breakfast recipes on pages 80–83. Later in the day, you are best off eating meals that contain protein- and fiber-rich foods to sustain more even blood-sugar levels.

root of your problem, in which case you will need to increase your intake of iron-rich foods (see the chart on pages 130–131) and even perhaps take iron supplements.

If your body is not detoxifying efficiently, you can raise your energy levels by changing to a diet that supports your body's detoxification mechanisms rather than hampering them (see pages 30–35). Alternatively, your tiredness could be the result of a sensitivity to certain foods (see pages 38–9). Again, simple dietary changes—identifying and eliminating from your diet the foods that are causing the adverse reaction—can make all the difference.

Common causes of persistent tiredness that are not directly diet-related include an underactive thyroid gland, which your doctor can test for. Lack of sleep is another obvious culprit—if you are not sleeping well, you are bound to be tired and tetchy. See pages 54–7 for advice on sleeping better. Depression (see pages 66–71) may also manifest itself as ongoing tiredness and irritability.

Eating for energy

The link between your diet and how energetic you feel is easy to see—after all, we know that if we drank a strong

KEY ENERGY NUTRIENTS

Nutrient	Rich food sources
Vitamin B1	Beef kidney and liver, brewer's yeast, brown rice, garbanzo beans, kidney beans, pork, rice bran, salmon, soybeans, sunflower seeds, wheatgerm, wholegrain wheat and rye
Vitamin B2	Almonds, brewer's yeast, cheese, chicken, mushrooms, wheatgerm
Vitamin B3	Beef liver, brewer's yeast, chicken, eggs, fish, sunflower seeds, turkey
Vitamin B5	Blue cheese, brewer's yeast, corn, eggs, lentils, liver, lobster, meats, peanuts, peas, soybeans, sunflower seeds, wheatgerm, wholegrain products
Vitamin B6	Avocados, bananas, bran, brewer's yeast, carrots, filberts, lentils, rice, salmon, shrimps, soybeans, sunflower seeds, tuna, walnuts, wheatgerm, wholegrain flour
Vitamin C	Blackcurrants, broccoli, Brussels sprouts, cabbage, collard greens, grapefruit, green peppers, guava, lemons, oranges, papaya, potatoes, spinach, strawberries, tomatoes, watercress
Chromium	Beef, brewer's yeast, chicken, eggs, fish, fruit, milk products, potatoes, whole grains
Coenzyme Q10	All foods, particularly beef, mackerel, sardines, soy oil, spinach
Magnesium	Almonds, fish, green leafy vegetables, kelp, molasses, nuts, soybeans, sunflower seeds, wheatgerm
Zinc	Egg yolk, fish, all meat, milk, molasses, oysters, sesame seeds, soybeans, sunflower seeds, turkey, wheatgerm, whole grains

ACTIVE INGREDIENT: B VITAMINS

Inside each cell in the body are minute energy factories called mitochondria. How much energy you feel you have and, to a large degree, your moods, depend on the production of energy inside every single one of these microscopic powerhouses. For energy to be created, a combustion process takes place. To fuel this process, the mitochondria require a constant supply of glucose, oxygen, and nutrients. Among the key nutrient players are vitamins B1, B3, B5, B6, and biotin (another B vitamin). B vitamins are also needed to help maintain healthy nerves and to produce the important neurotransmitters (brain messenger molecules) that help maintain mood and control appetite.

When we are under stress, we tend to eat a diet high in refined foods (from which much of the B-vitamin content has been removed). So, although the demand for B vitamins is higher, we are not necessarily meeting this increased need. It is therefore important to include plenty of foods that are rich in B vitamins in your diet. Particularly good sources of B vitamins include: brewer's yeast, brown rice and other whole grains, sunflower seeds, wheatgerm, nuts, eggs, fish, lean meat, and poultry (see also the chart on page 45).

However, increasing your B-vitamin supplies is only part of the story: It is also important to minimize your intake of refined foods, which have been depleted of the B vitamins and other nutrients nature provided them with. For example, refined flour contains less than a quarter of the levels of vitamin B1 and a fifth of the B3 found in its wholegrain counterpart. You should also try to steer clear of the substances that hamper the absorption and use of some B vitamins in the body. Alcohol, caffeine, and some drugs, including the contraceptive pill, are all culprits.

In addition to eating a diet rich in fresh, whole foods and avoiding refined foods, taking a B-complex vitamin supplement (or a multi that is high in B vitamins) can help ensure that you are getting enough of these important nutrients. Do remember, though, that supplements are not a substitute for eating well, cutting out stimulants, and getting enough sleep. Recipes that are rich in B vitamins include:

BREAKFASTS: Very Berry Breaky (page 83); Designer Muesli (page 83)

LIGHT MEAL: Baby Spinach and Goat's Cheese Salad (page 84)

MAIN MEALS: Frittata (page 100); Lentils with Spinach (page 110)

DESSERT: Khosaf (page 121)

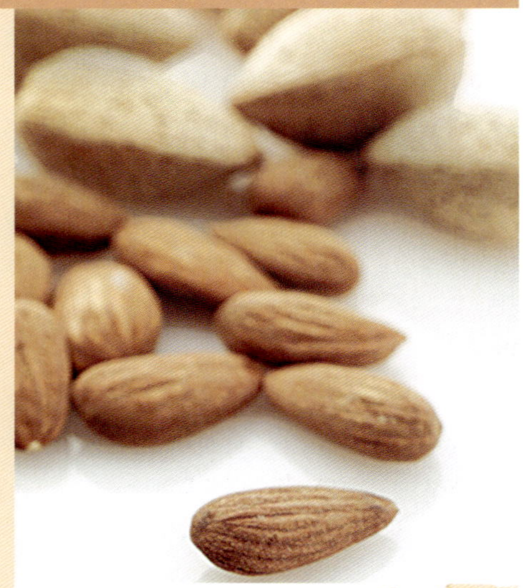

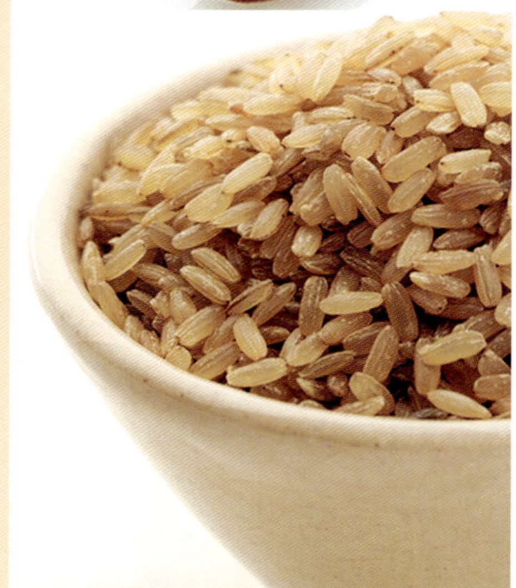

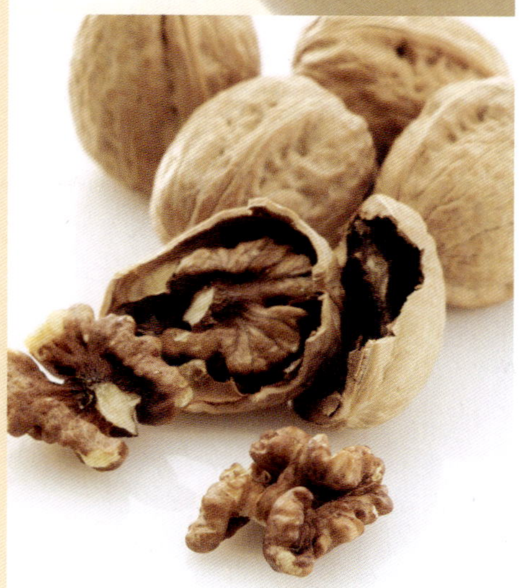

coffee and ate a bar of chocolate, we would be buzzing, for a while at least. On a cellular level, we are, with our diets, literally fueling all our cells to produce energy through a carefully controlled chemical reaction. The type of fuel we use correlates to our performance, much like that of a car. In fact, many people are probably more careful about fueling and servicing their car than they are their own body.

To produce energy, each cell needs a supply of fuel in the form of glucose, derived from the carbohydrates and sugars that we eat. There's little danger of any of us not getting enough carbohydrates, but the process of converting the fuel into energy requires a range of micro-nutrients. The best way to provide your body with all these nutrients is to eat a varied diet of fresh, unprocessed foods. See the chart on page 45 for a list of foods that are rich in energy-boosting nutrients, and pages 22–5 for more on a nutrient-rich diet. It can also help to take vitamin and mineral supplements, but it is important to remember that they are just that—supplements to, not substitutes for, a good diet (see page 128).

Avoiding foods that sap your energy is just as important as eating energy-rich foods. The energy drainers are generally foods and drinks—and especially stimulants, such as coffee, alcohol, and candy—that play havoc with our blood-sugar levels (for more on the mechanism controlling blood-sugar levels, see pages 12–17).

Breaking the dependency

Especially when we are feeling constantly exhausted, we often become addicted to stimulating "superfuel" foods and drinks to keep us going (see the box on page 69 for a list of common stimulants). Unfortunately, these can give us only a very temporary boost, followed by a dive in mood and energy that leaves us reaching for the next stimulant. Meanwhile, we require ever-larger doses to produce the desired temporary buzz. Harsh as it may sound, the best way to stop the seesawing of energy and moods is to give up stimulants altogether.

Coffee—friend or foe?

Coffee can certainly give you a buzz but, like many "addictive" substances, the initial high is inevitably followed by a low—in effect, a withdrawal symptom. It is no coincidence that coffee drinkers often sleep less soundly than non-coffee drinkers. Apart from playing havoc with your adrenal glands (see page 18), coffee is also a diuretic, so it can leave you dehydrated, which can also make you tired and short-tempered. Nor is decaffeinated coffee a viable alternative; not only does it still contain other natural stimulants, such as theophylline and threobromine, but it may also contain residues of harsh chemicals used in the decaffeinating process.

You do not necessarily have to give up coffee entirely—just cutting back can help your energy levels to recover. For some people, this may mean cutting down from six daily coffees to one or two; for others, it means going from two to none. If you find this hard, I suggest you try not to have a coffee or tea before at least 11am, so that you are not relying on a stimulant to kick-start your day. As you begin to reduce your intake, you may feel even more tired or headachey. This is perfectly normal, and not a good reason to start up again. If you are following the other guidelines in this book for maintaining even blood-sugar levels and eating a balanced, nutritious diet to help boost your energy and maintain even moods, you should find you no longer "need" so many doses of caffeine.

ENERGY-BOOSTING RECIPES

BREAKFASTS: Scrambled Eggs on Rye with Leeks and Mushrooms (page 80); Buckwheat Crêpes (page 83)

LIGHT MEALS: Nanna's Rice Salad (page 88); Spicy Bean Salad (page 89); Chunky Vegetable Soup (page 94); Leek and Potato Soup (page 97)

MAIN MEALS: Kebabs (page 102); Broiled Mackerel on a Bed of Stinging Nettles (page 105); Sweet Roast Lamb (page 109); Seatown Kedgeree (page 109); Shiitake Roast Chicken (page 110)

DESSERTS: Baked Bananas with Raspberry Sauce (page 121); Crunchy Oaty Crumble (page 121)

Countless women experience premenstrual syndrome, and many believe its unpleasant symptoms are unavoidable. However, for most sufferers, a combination of simple dietary changes, appropriate nutritional supplements, and regular exercise can make PMS a thing of the past.

premenstrual problems

On the list below, tick the symptoms that are familiar and persistent for you in the days leading up to your period:

- ☐ chocolate, sugar, and carbohydrate cravings
- ☐ overeating
- ☐ water retention, puffiness, bloating
- ☐ mood swings
- ☐ irritability
- ☐ despair or a sense of insecurity
- ☐ feeling tearful or anxious
- ☐ tender breasts
- ☐ clumsiness or forgetfulness
- ☐ excessive tiredness

If you regularly experience any of the above symptoms in the 10 days or so before your period, only to find they miraculously disappear once your period has started, then it is likely that you have premenstrual syndrome, or PMS. For many women, this slide into misery is an all-too familiar part of their monthly cycle and entails anything from three days to two weeks of discomfort and upset.

PMS is difficult to define, for it affects women in a wide range of ways for different lengths of time and is caused by a complex variety of factors. Because PMS is so common (one US study concluded that up to 40 percent of women who menstruate experience some PMS symptoms), even extreme symptoms are sometimes dismissed as normal or inevitable. Yet most women who suffer from PMS say that it adversely effects their relationships with family, friends, and co-workers. Although the causes of PMS are often mixed, factors known to be linked to the syndrome include hormonal and blood-sugar imbalance, poor nutrient status, and stress.

Hormonal balance

The most significant culprit behind most cases of PMS is hormonal imbalance. It is widely thought that many women with PMS suffer from an imbalance in the ratio between the main female hormones: estrogen and progesterone. Too much estrogen in relation to progesterone seems to be particularly at fault, and is believed to be most pronounced in women whose main premenstrual symptoms are anxiety, irritability, and mood swings. Excess estrogen can be caused by various factors, including exposure to estrogen-like chemicals in the environment (see box, page 51) and poor digestion, detoxification, and elimination.

The liver (see page 33) plays a vital role in recycling and breaking down hormones. If, for any reason, your liver is not working quite up to scratch, you can end up with too much estrogen. The liver may be overloaded by an excess of alcohol, drugs, coffee, fatty meats, and dairy products, an

BITE-SIZE SOLUTION

To help reduce water retention and bloating in the days leading up to your period, try to cut out all added salt from your diet and reduce your consumption of foods with a high salt content, such as potato chips, hams, and ready meals.

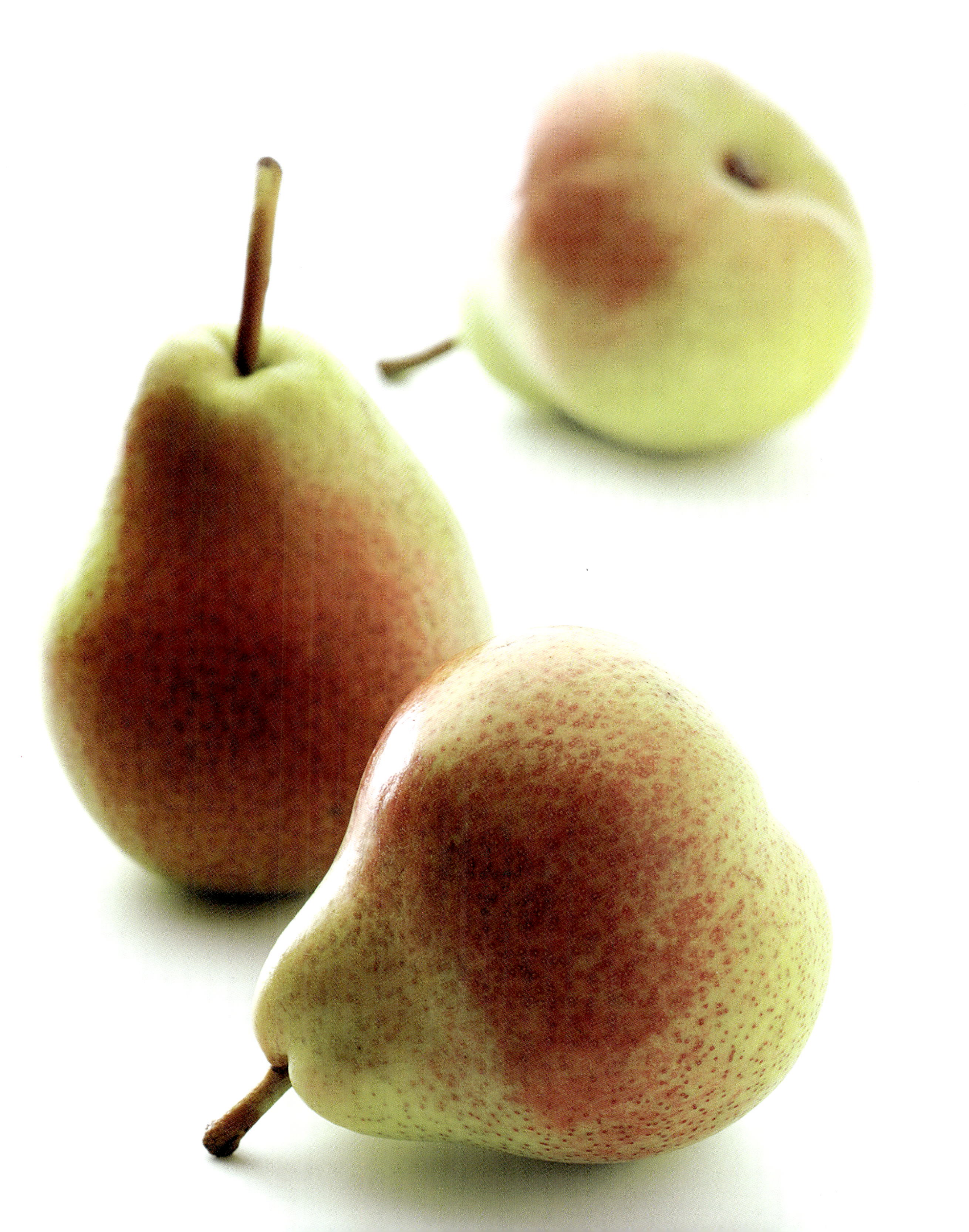

unhealthy digestive system, or even a lack of certain nutrients such as B vitamins (see box, page 46), which are needed for the breakdown of estrogen. Some women—especially those who suffer from irritability, depression, and insomnia—see dramatic reductions in their PMS symptoms when they ease the burden on their liver simply by giving up coffee. Excess estrogen can also remain in the body if it is not being eliminated properly, particularly if your digestion is not good or you are often constipated. One of the main ways of encouraging your body to eliminate optimally is to make sure you are regularly eating naturally fiber-rich foods, such as fresh fruit and vegetables, beans, lentils, and whole grains (see pages 30–37). You can also help to correct your hormonal balance by increasing your intake of foods that are rich in phyto-estrogens (see box, opposite).

RECIPES TO COMBAT PMS

BREAKFAST: Filling Fruit Bowl (page 80); Very Berry Breaky (page 83); Designer Muesli (page 83)
LIGHT MEALS: Mongettes Charentaises (page 91); Japanese-Style Tuna Salad (page 92); Puy Lentil Salad (page 93); Fish Soup Provençale (page 97); Bean and Zucchini Soup (page 98); Tabouleh (page 114; pictured)
MAIN MEALS: Trout with Sunflower Seeds (page 104); Salmon Rolls (page 106); Spiced Bean Stew (page 113)
DESSERTS: Baked Bananas with Raspberry Sauce (page 121); Khosaf (page 121)

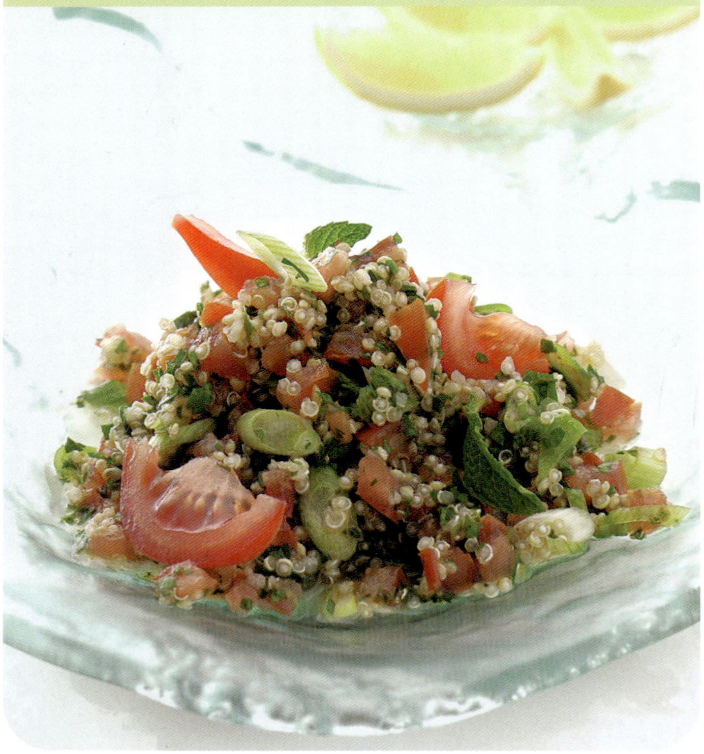

Blood-sugar balance

Women whose blood-sugar levels seesaw throughout the month, resulting in mood and energy swings over the course of each day, usually find that these symptoms are exacerbated in the lead-up to their period. If you experience cravings for starchy, sweet, or fatty foods before you menstruate, blood-sugar imbalance is probably to blame. It is usually helpful to take steps to maintain even blood-sugar levels throughout the month (see pages 12–17) in order to reduce the chances of extreme versions of these symptoms surfacing in the pre-menstrual phase. For more on food cravings, see pages 58–9.

Supportive supplements

There are several key nutrients that can help reduce the symptoms that you experience before a period. In addition to a healthy diet that is low in sugar, refined foods, fatty foods, coffee, salt, and alcohol, some nutritional supplements can provide significant relief.

As many as 80 percent of women with PMS have been found to have low supplies of the mineral magnesium. Crucial for countless functions in the body that may contribute to controlling PMS, magnesium is found in almonds, fish, green leafy vegetables, molasses, nuts, soybeans, sunflower seeds, and wheatgerm. For a particularly effective remedy, it's best to take a daily magnesium supplement at a dose of 6 mg per 2.2 lb of body weight.

Magnesium appears to work synergistically with the vitamin B6, which many women also find helps relieve PMS. It is best not to take individual B vitamins alone, as they work alongside one another. Instead, take a high-strength multivitamin that contains at least 50 mg of B6 as well as the spectrum of B vitamins and other nutrients.

ACTIVE INGREDIENT: PHYTO-ESTROGENS

The delicate balance between the estrogen and progesterone in your body can be disturbed by exposure to many man-made chemicals, such as pharmaceuticals (for example, drugs), agrochemicals (including pesticides and fertilizers), and petrochemicals (such as plastics). These chemicals contain toxic xeno-estrogens ("xeno" means external), which can act similarly to strong estrogens in the body, worsening PMS symptoms, as well as other problems, including endometriosis and infertility.

If you suffer from PMS, you should try to minimize your exposure to these harmful chemicals—not always an easy task. Fortunately, there are other ways of helping to nudge estrogen levels back into balance. Scientists have discovered that some plants contain substances known as phyto-estrogens ("phyto" means plant), which can help to block the effects of excess estrogen in the body, evening out any imbalance in the ratio between estrogen and progesterone.

Phyto-estrogens appear to work by locking into the estrogen-receptor sites on cells—in doing so they block out the stronger xeno-estrogens. At the same time, if a woman is actually low in estrogen—as can occur during the menopause, for example—phyto-estrogens act as a weak estrogen. They thereby help relieve the woman's symptoms by boosting estrogen levels while still blocking out the harmful xeno-estrogens.

It is therefore helpful for many women with PMS, and also for women suffering from menopausal symptoms, to include some phyto-estrogens in their diet. For example, eating some soy produce three or four times a week can be extremely beneficial, as soy is a particularly rich source of estrogen. Phyto-estrogens are also found in citrus fruits, oats, fennel, alfalfa, licorice, celery, flaxseeds, beans, sesame, rice bran, wheatgerm, peas, carrots, apples, and pears. Herbs that are good sources of phyto-estrogens include sage, parsley, and basil.

The following recipes are rich in phyto-estrogens:

BREAKFASTS: High-Five Seeds sprinkled on yogurt or cereal (page 82); Designer Muesli (page 83)

LIGHT MEALS: Houmous, Avocado, and Alfalfa baked-potato topping (page 86); Spicy Bean Salad (page 89)

MAIN MEALS: Lentils with Spinach (page 110)

DESSERTS: Crunchy Oaty Crumble (page 121)

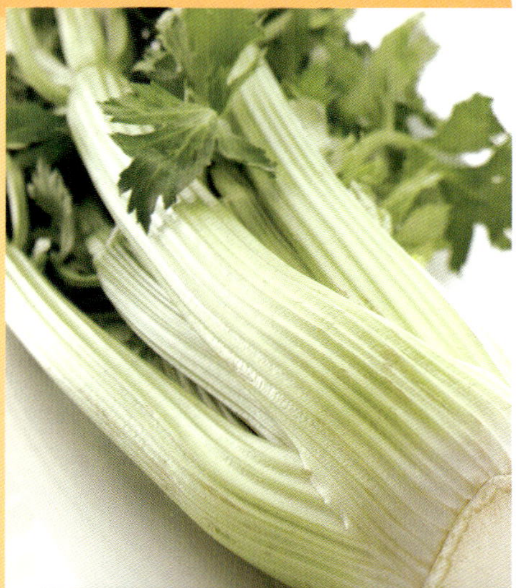

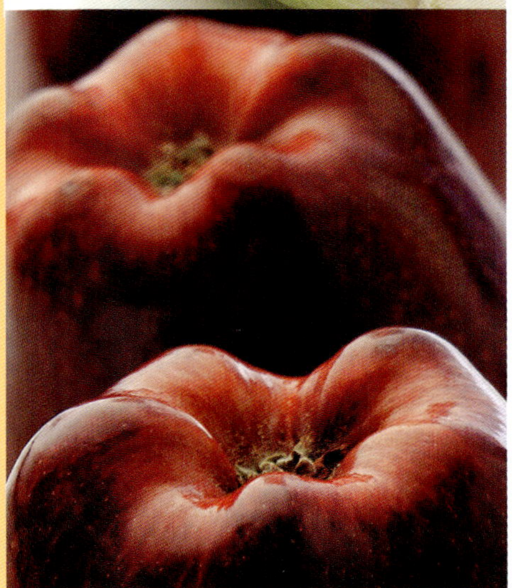

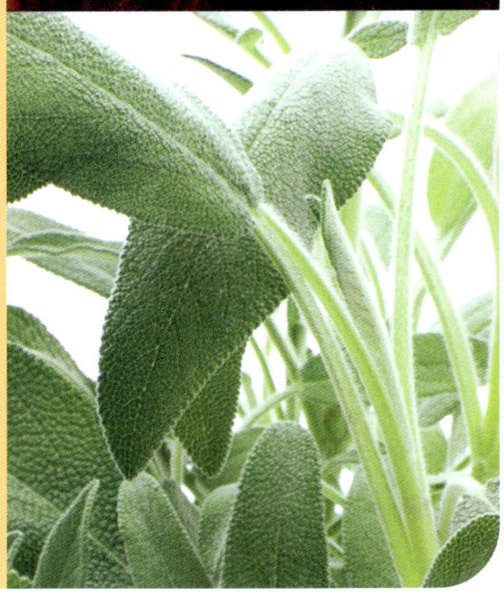

As much as 10 percent of the population in the US experience what is known as seasonal affective disorder (SAD), or winter depression—a change in mood, energy, and appetite that sets in with the coming of the long, dark winter days and is relieved only by the start of spring.

winter woes: SAD

On the list below, tick the symptoms that are familiar and persistent for you in the winter months:

- ☐ increased sleep
- ☐ feeling unrefreshed after sleep
- ☐ craving starchy and sweet foods
- ☐ overeating
- ☐ weight gain
- ☐ feelings of hopelessness
- ☐ irritability
- ☐ anxiety
- ☐ inability to concentrate
- ☐ lethargy, lack of motivation

If you ticked five or more symptoms, you may suffer from SAD. To most of us, shorter days herald the imminent cosiness of winter. But for people who have SAD, the onset of fall brings a dread of the miserable times to come.

Governed by hormones, our body's internal rhythms control behavior patterns such as sleep, energy, and appetite. For most of us, our daily activities are rarely aligned with the way we were designed to live—we do not usually sleep when it gets dark, awaken when it is light, and eat regular, healthy meals that maintain even blood-sugar levels when we feel hungry. By living out of synch with our natural patterns, we disturb delicate rhythms, which can, in sensitive people, result in disorders such as SAD. However, by using similar strategies to those suggested for dealing with depression (see pages 66–71), there is much you can do nutritionally to ease SAD symptoms.

Isn't SAD just depression?

The criteria used to diagnose SAD, as opposed to clinical depression, lie in the timing—a person with winter depression may, even without treatment, feel much better in the spring time. And, unlike classically depressed people, who are often affected by insomnia, most SAD sufferers experience extreme tiredness and sleep more than usual. They also tend to have a significant increase in appetite and weight during the winter months.

If you are experiencing severe winter depression, you should consult your doctor.

Food cravings

Some substances in the body have been shown to have a particularly significant impact on seasonal changes in mood, energy, and appetite. One such substance is the neurotransmitter serotonin, low levels of which have been shown to be responsible for mood disorders in general.

The precise way in which serotonin affects SAD sufferers has not yet been demonstrated, but the theory of a link is reinforced by the carbohydrate (starch and sugar) cravings that people with SAD experience. Serotonin is in part responsible for determining our appetite—when serotonin levels are low, we feel more hungry. Carbohydrate-rich foods trigger the production of serotonin, so SAD sufferers are, perhaps subconsciously, reaching for more bread, pasta, cereal, cakes, candy, and other starchy foods in order to help regulate their moods and boost their energy. If you have SAD, there is nothing wrong with eating starchy

A RAY OF HOPE

The control centers in our brains that determine our moods and daily rhythms are governed in part by the amount of light that enters our eyes. When light hits certain parts of the retina, it effects the release of the hormone melatonin. During the night, or in darkness, melatonin production increases, making us sleepy. When day breaks and our eyes are exposed to natural light, melatonin production stops. During the dark winter days, therefore, the control mechanism for melatonin release changes. It appears that SAD sufferers are especially sensitive to this change.

Light- or phototherapy is a treatment for SAD involving daily exposure to high-intensity, broad-spectrum artifical light from a light box, thus suppressing the production of melatonin. Phototherapy may also help to increase levels of the mood-boosting neurotransmitter serotonin. Several research trials have now shown that light therapy is an effective treatment for winter depression, although 20 percent of SAD sufferers do not appear to benefit from light therapy alone.

foods to improve your mood, as long as you are able to stick to unrefined, wholesome carbohydrates, such as muesli, brown rice, a wholegrain-bread sandwich, or an oaty fruit bar, and you really do feel much better for some time after eating it. Very sugary, refined foods, such as cookies, doughnuts, and candy, are best avoided as these are likely to stimulate weight gain and increase cravings.

Serotonin is produced in the body from the amino acid (protein constituent) tryptophan. Eating foods that are rich in tryptophan, such as chicken, turkey, milk, yogurt, bananas, figs, tuna, seaweed, and sunflower seeds, can help your body create more serotonin. See the box on page 70 for details on how to raise your levels of tryptophan.

Some research has shown that people with SAD who eat more carbohydrates also respond better to light therapy (see box, left), so combining a light treatment with methods designed to increase serotonin levels may be the most effective way of combating winter depression.

Levels of another neurotransmitter, dopamine, have been found to increase when bright light hits the back of the eye. As dopamine is thought to improve alertness and concentration, reduced levels in darker months could well contribute to the lethargy and low moods characteristic of SAD. Certain foods can help raise dopamine levels—try to include in your diet lean meat, dairy products, fish, and eggs, all of which are good sources of an amino acid called phenylalanine, which the body can convert into dopamine.

Balancing blood sugar

In order to relieve the common symptoms of SAD—not just low moods and energy, but also increased appetite—you need to eat plenty of foods that help balance blood-sugar levels (see pages 12–17). The chart of fast- and slow-releasing carbohydrates on page 16 gives you clear guidelines on eating for sustained energy rather than quick bursts. Other ways of doing this include: Eating three meals a day and, if necessary, a couple of snacks in between; having protein- and fiber-rich foods with each meal; and avoiding substances such as coffee, alcohol, sugar, and cigarettes, which play havoc with blood-sugar levels. The mineral chromium can help reduce cravings for very sweet, starchy foods—take 100 mcg at breakfast and at lunch.

RECIPES TO EASE SAD

BREAKFASTS: Apple Oatmeal (page 82); Designer Muesli (page 83); Poached Eggs with Asparagus (page 83)

LIGHT MEALS: Chicken and Mushroom Pâté (page 87); Bean and Zucchini Soup (page 98)

MAIN MEALS: Stuffed Vegetables (page 100); Frittata (page 100); Broiled Swordfish in Caper Salsa (page 102); Thai-style Icefish (page 106); Sweet Roast Lamb (page 109);

DESSERTS: Apricot Ice Cream with Pistachios (page 118); Tropical Whizz (page 122); Fireside Pears (page 122)

Modern living is not generally a recipe for good sleep, or enough of it. Yet most people cannot function well on much less than seven hours of uninterrupted sleep a night. Sleeplessness not only leaves you feeling exhausted but can also end up dampening your moods.

sleepless nights

On the list below, tick the symptoms that are familiar and persistent for you:

- ☐ difficulty getting to sleep
- ☐ waking up in the night
- ☐ waking early and not getting back to sleep
- ☐ feeling unrefreshed after a night's sleep
- ☐ putting off going to bed, even when tired
- ☐ energy slumps/dozing during the day
- ☐ falling asleep early in the evening but not sleeping well at night

If you ticked four or more symptoms, you could probably benefit from altering your diet and lifestyle in order to improve the quality and amount of sleep you are getting. An ongoing sleeplessness problem can affect productivity and relationships. Without adequate sleep, the body quickly shows clear signs of stress. Sleep deprivation makes us tired, moody, and irritable and, in the long term, even depressed. Sleep-deprived individuals have also been found to have a reduction in the immune cells needed to resist invaders, reducing their ability to fight off illness and infection.

Sleep is made up of a series of regular sleep cycles of varying lengths and depths. In the average, healthy person, the whole sleep cycle, including stage four (the deepest kind of sleep), lasts roughly 90 minutes. The first two complete sleep cycles are thought to contain mostly stage three and four sleep; REM (dream sleep) occurs mainly in the second half of the sleep period; and lighter sleep (stages one and two) comes only at the end of the night. If you are deprived of sleep for a while, at the earliest opportunity your body will try to make up this deficit by quickly going to stage four and REM sleep in each cycle.

Sleeplessness is a condition that occurs when, over a period of time (usually at night), a person wants to sleep but is unable to. Insomnia, on the other hand, describes a condition that occurs when someone who has previously been a good sleeper suffers from chronic sleeplessness that lasts for several weeks or longer.

This section explores how you can overcome sleeplessness and improve your sleep through dietary methods. If you are suffering from insomnia you should see your doctor or other healthcare practitioner, or contact an organization that specializes in sleep problems. Remember that insomnia can be a symptom of chronic anxiety, depression or stress rather than the cause, and will often disappear if other problems are dealt with.

The chemistry of sleep

Many of our body's daily rhythms, including those that dictate our energy and sleepiness, are finely tuned mechanisms that depend on certain hormonal patterns, body chemicals, and nutrients. At night time, levels of the hormone cortisol should dip, calming your body and preparing it for sleep. If, however, your cortisol levels are out of kilter for any reason (usually owing to stress or a diet high in stimulants or sugar), your ability to get to sleep, to sleep through the night, or to wake up refreshed is likely to be impaired. If cortisol levels are high at night, this suppresses

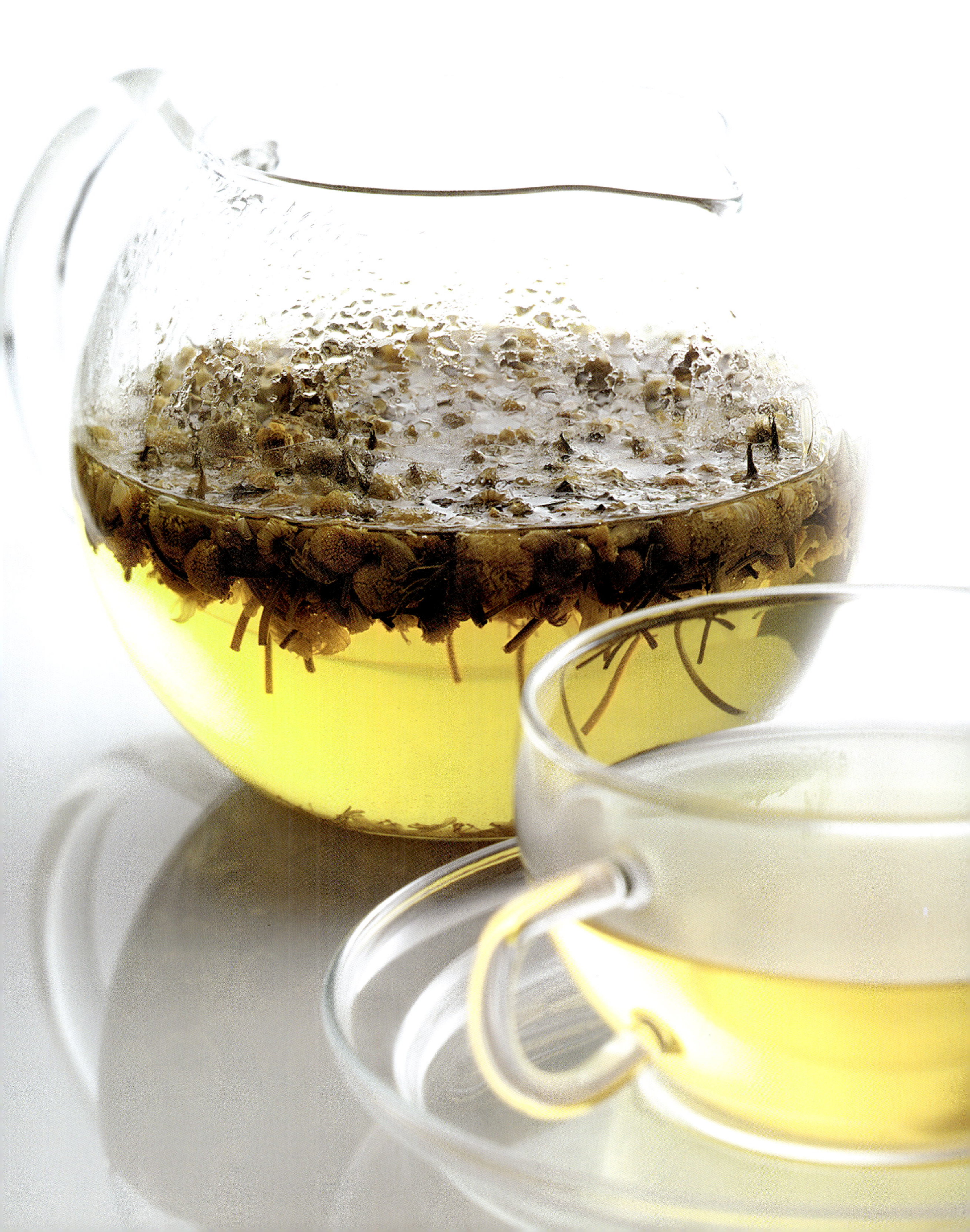

SOLVING YOUR SLEEP PROBLEMS

One or several of the following could be keeping you from getting a good night's sleep. Cast your eye down the list of problems and their solutions to see which you could be dealing with in order to sleep better:

- Eating too close to bedtime: If your body is busy digesting a recent meal, your sleep will be disturbed. Eat at least three hours before going to bed.
- Excessive/late caffeine or alcohol intake: This raises cortisol levels, which keeps you awake. Avoid drinking caffeine or alcohol, at least from early evening onward.
- Late cigarette smoking: This raises cortisol levels. Avoid smoking, at least from early evening onward.
- Indigestion: The discomfort this causes is likely to prevent you from sleeping well. Eat early in the evening, slowly, and in moderation.
- Widely fluctuating blood-sugar levels: Dips in blood sugar during the night may wake you up. See pages 12–17 for advice on balancing blood-sugar levels.

the release of growth hormones, which are essential for daily tissue repair and growth. A nutritionist can run a saliva test for you to determine whether your cortisol rhythm is out of synch. See pages 18–21 for advice on improving your diet to support your adrenals and regulate cortisol production.

Food and sleeplessness

If you are overeating or eating high amounts of starchy or fatty foods, or very refined, sugary foods that stress your body, you are more likely to feel sluggish and lethargic, for these foods place high demands on your digestive processes. Unfortunately, feeling sluggish during the day is rarely followed by a good night's sleep. A high intake of stimulants such as coffee, tea, alcohol (as well as cigarettes and recreational drugs), especially close to bedtime, will interfere with either your ability to get to sleep or your sleep pattern during the night.

Some natural health practitioners also suggest avoiding foods such as pork, cheese, chocolate, eggplants, tomatoes, potatoes, and wine near bedtime as they are rich in an amino acid called tyramine, which the body can convert to norepinephrine, a brain stimulant.

The serotonin–sleep link

Another body chemical that is linked to the ability to sleep well is serotonin, a neurotransmitter made in the body from the amino acid tryptophan (see box, page 70). Eating foods rich in tryptophan—such as bananas, chicken, figs, milk, seaweed, sunflower seeds, tuna, turkey, and yogurt—can help induce sleepiness.

If you eat supper early, you may be tempted to have a nibble before going to bed. The following snacks are rich in tryptophan and should therefore help you sleep:

- oat or rice cakes with houmous/cottage cheese or a slice of chicken/turkey, or with tuna
- oat or rice cakes with tahini and a little honey or nut butter
- a small pot of natural yogurt with sunflower seeds/ chopped dates or figs/bananas
- banana milkshake (with milk or soy milk)
- piece of fruit and a handful of sunflower seeds or almonds
- a couple of dried dates and a few sunflower seeds or almonds

For women—the cycle of sleeplessness

Many women find that how long and deeply they sleep varies with their menstrual cycle; sleeplessness is particularly common just before a period or during the menopause. Because estrogen influences the production of brain chemicals that keep you alert, and progesterone can trigger sleepiness, it is not surprising that hormonal fluctuations cause sleep variations. Although you cannot necessarily keep your hormones under control, if you know when you are likely to experience sleeplessness you can take extra precautions to help you sleep. Perhaps it is no coincidence that nutrients that are useful for relieving PMS (see pages 48–51), such as vitamin B6 and magnesium, can also help with sleep difficulties.

Nutrients for sleep

Sleep difficulties can be triggered or exacerbated by a lack of the minerals calcium and magnesium, because they work together to calm the body and help relax muscles. Your diet is more likely to be low in magnesium than calcium, so make sure you are eating plenty of magnesium-rich foods, such as seeds, nuts, green vegetables, whole grains, and seafood (see also the chart on pages 130–131). Having some magnesium in the evening, perhaps even in a supplement, may also help. Milk products, green vegetables, nuts, seafood, and molasses are particularly good sources of calcium. Ensuring you are getting adequate B vitamins helps support the body in many ways, including boosting its ability to deal with stress. However, take B-complex vitamins early in the day rather than in the evening as they are also involved in energy production.

Natural nightcaps

Sleep aids of any kind are unlikely to provide much benefit if it is other underlying factors that are keeping you awake at night. If you're eating badly, drinking a lot of coffee or alcohol, or are particularly stressed, you need to resolve those issues first. It's really best to use sleep aids—whether natural or pharmaceutical—as a last resort when you have exhausted all the other solutions mentioned in this section.

Medical sedatives are generally bad news in that they are usually addictive. As your tolerance of them increases, you need to take ever higher doses to feel any effect. They can trigger a range of side effects, including daytime drowsiness, memory problems, confusion, depression, dry mouth, sluggishness, and all sorts of other unpleasant symptoms. Medical sedatives are also strong chemicals that need to be detoxified by the body, placing a burden on your liver.

There are many non-addictive natural substances that can help you sleep, although they should be used only occasionally. Valerian, hops, passionflower, oats, and lemon balm (melissa) are all herbs that have a long history of use as sedatives. Combinations of such herbs are available in most healthfood stores and pharmacies. Some herbs make pleasant hot drinks—chamomile is particularly well known for its calming properties, and makes a good pre-bedtime drink as a tea or infusion (pictured, page 55).

RECIPES FOR IMPROVED SLEEP

You are more likely to sleep well if you eat your main meal at lunchtime and have a lighter meal in the early evening.

LIGHT MEALS: Baby Spinach and Goat's Cheese Salad (page 84); Smoked Fish Pâté (page 87); Dahl (page 90); Mongettes Charentaises (page 91); Thai-Style Noodle Soup (page 96); Fish Soup Provençale (page 97); Bean and Zucchini Soup (page 98)

MAIN MEALS: Stuffed Vegetables (page 100); Broiled Swordfish in Caper Salsa (page 102); Sesame Stir-Fry (page 106); Gobble Pie (page 109); Shiitake Roast Chicken (page 110; pictured); Spiced Bean Stew (page 113); Quinoa with Roast Vegetables (page 113)

DESSERTS: Apricot Ice Cream with Pistachios (page 118); Baked Bananas with Raspberry Sauce (page 121)

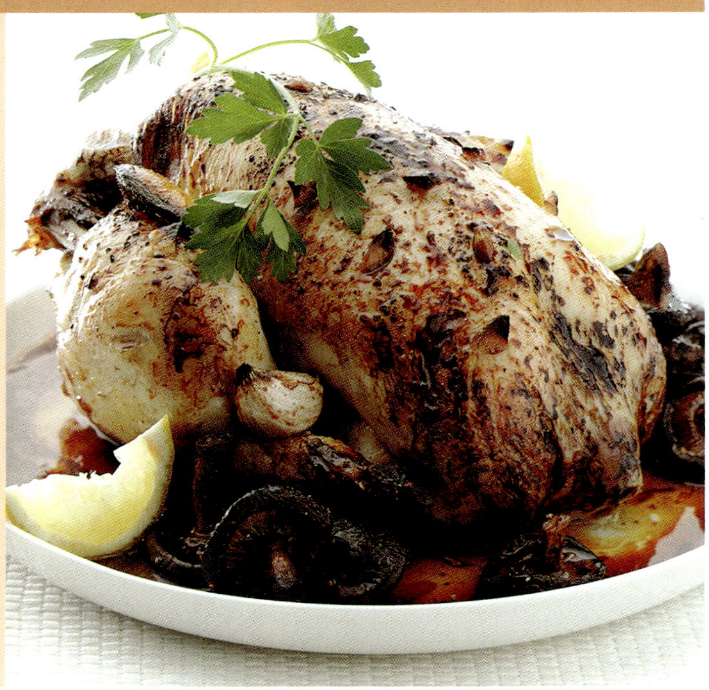

Increasing numbers of people—especially young women—are reporting that their appetite and eating patterns are out of control. While it is not unusual to turn to food when you are feeling low, if comfort eating becomes uncontrolled bingeing, your health can be threatened.

binge eating

On the list below, tick the symptoms that are familiar and persistent for you:

- ☐ feeling that your eating is "out of control"
- ☐ recurrent episodes of binge eating
- ☐ eating large amounts of food quickly, even when not feeling hungry
- ☐ hiding food (or evidence such as wrappers)
- ☐ eating until you feel uncomfortably full
- ☐ feelings of disgust or guilt during and after overeating
- ☐ binge eating triggered by uncomfortable feelings such as anger, anxiety, or shame
- ☐ disgust or embarrassment about body size
- ☐ feelings of worthlessness
- ☐ mood swings and irritability

If you ticked five or more of the above symptoms, you may be suffering from disturbed eating patterns.

Some people can open a packet of chocolate-chip cookies, take a couple, and put the packet away. For others, this is inconceivable—they cannot resist the urge to eat the whole packet in one sitting. Food cravings and overeating are often linked to mood problems such as PMS, SAD, stress, and depression, as well as feelings of loneliness, anxiety, or boredom. It is no coincidence that people tend to turn to food for comfort when they are feeling low, for certain foods trigger chemical reactions in the body that bring some temporary relief. The danger is that occasional comfort eating can turn into a highly destructive pattern of regular, compulsive overeating that is notoriously hard to break.

Binge-eating disorder

Sometimes also referred to as compulsive overeating, binge-eating disorder (BED) is characterized by frequent episodes of uncontrolled overeating. Unlike bulimics, BED sufferers do not purge themselves after bingeing, and therefore tend to put on weight. A person of any age, sex, or size may suffer from compulsive overeating. Statistics show that many people who experience BED have a history of depression, and that 30 percent of the women who seek help for weight loss are suffering from BED. Dieting appears to cause a sense of deprivation—as well as starvation and low blood sugar—which can easily result in bingeing.

Tackling compulsive overeating

In combating any kind of compulsive eating disorder, the most successful results are achieved through a combination of psychological and physiological approaches. That is, the patient examines and deals with the emotions that trigger overeating and takes nutritional measures to curb the cravings. The aim of this book is to explore the physiological causes of mood disorders and to propose nutritional solutions. For

BITE-SIZE SOLUTION

To stave off that mid-afternoon craving, avoid having a heavy, carbohydrate-rich lunch. Instead of a sandwich or baked potato, have a large salad with a good-sized portion of chicken, fish, or cheese.

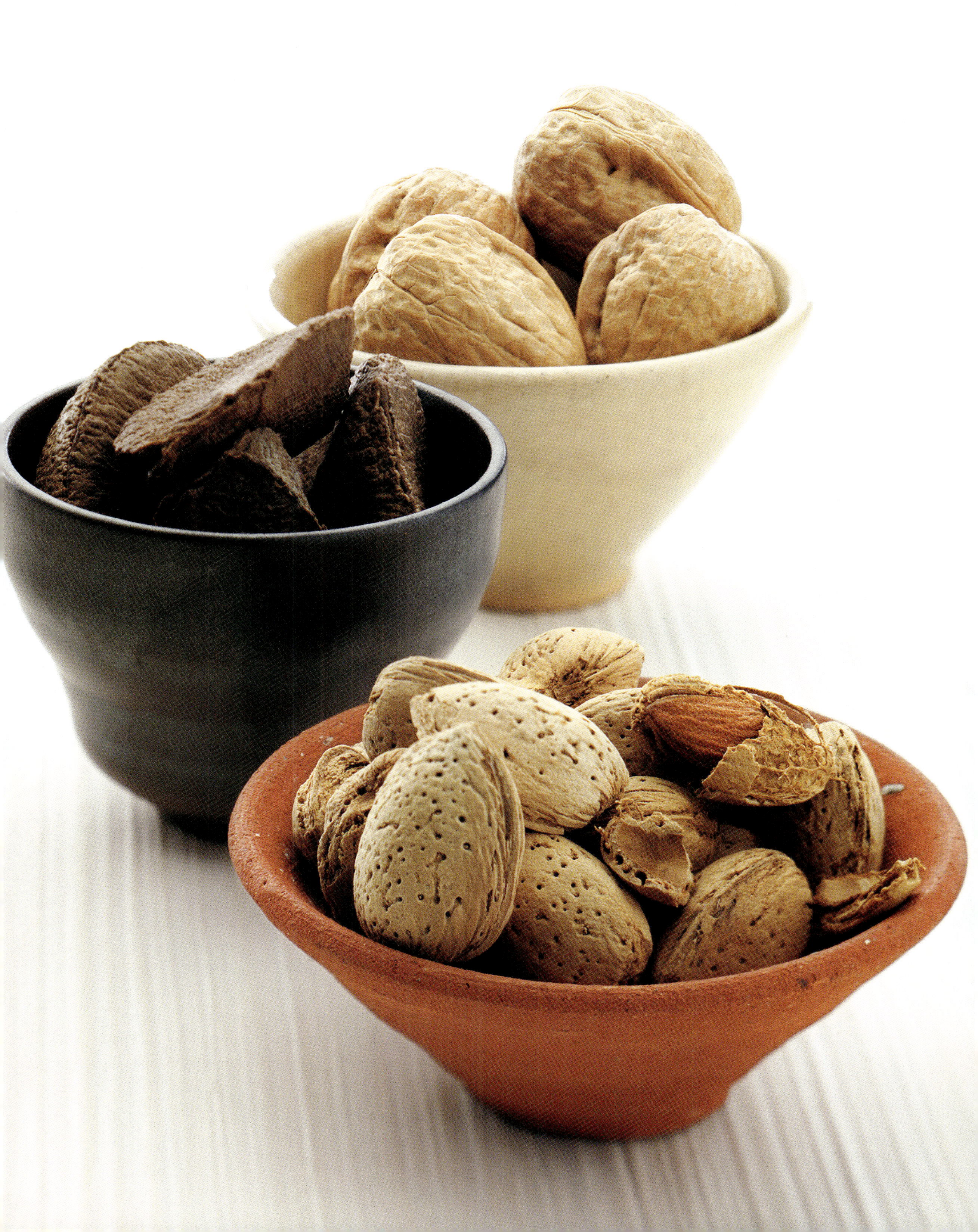

CHOCOLATE—SINNER OR SAVIOR?

Anyone with a sweet tooth or compulsive food cravings knows that sometimes nothing but chocolate will do. Chocolate has been scientifically shown to have in-built feel-good factors, including mental stimulants such as caffeine and theobromine. The sugar in chocolate helps increase blood-sugar levels, which give your energy and mood a boost. Combined with fat, the sugar is also believed to release endorphins, or feel-good chemicals, in the brain. Chocolate is a source of the energy mineral magnesium too, low levels of which are linked to premenstrual symptoms. Given all these stimulating effects, it is no surprise that chocolate is tempting—and addictive.

While the high levels of sugar, saturated fats, hydrogenated fats, and other additives in chocolate are clearly not desirable for good health in large amounts, there is certainly no harm in having a little chocolate sometimes. The challenge for a person who tends to binge is how to have a little without succumbing to a lot more. It can sometimes be best to allow yourself a small amount of chocolate in order to satisfy the craving. I recommend buying just a small bar of good-quality, dark chocolate (preferably organic), which has a strong, sweet taste and is most likely to answer the "need."

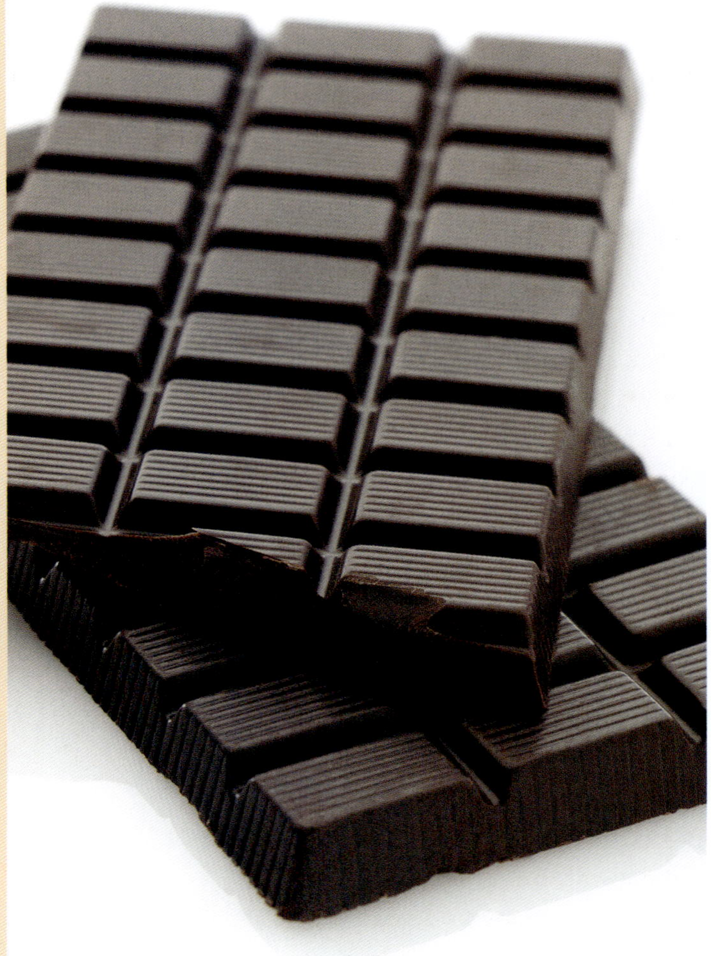

more on talking therapies that can help you to resolve the emotional problems behind your disturbed eating patterns, see pages 134–5.

Whatever may have been the initial trigger for the first "attack" of compulsive bingeing, it is imbalances in the body's chemistry linked to appetite, mood, and energy that contribute to sustaining the disorder.

Appetite control

The body has natural impulses that signal hunger and satisfaction with a meal. However, in some people this messaging system is ignored or becomes unbalanced as a result of an eating disorder. One hormone in particular—cholecystokinin (CCK)—aids the digestive process and is also known to give the sign that you are full after a certain amount of food. However, partly as a result of extreme over- or undereating, people who binge appear to have either low levels of CCK or a dulled response to it.

It is very important to sit down to eat, eat slowly, and chew well. CCK is released as food enters the small intestine from the stomach. If you eat slowly, the hormone is released and the satiety message is received while you are still eating. If, on the other hand, you wolf down your food, the satiety message is not passed on until you have finished eating, by which time it is too late to receive the signal that you have eaten enough.

Seeking serotonin

As with many disorders linked to mood, people who eat compulsively have also been found to have low levels of the feel-good neurotransmitter serotonin. (One scientific study found that antidepressant medication that raises serotonin levels is effective at reducing the incidence of binges.)

It is not by chance that you are more likely to crave sweet or starchy foods such as chocolate, cookies, or bread if you feel low. When we eat such foods they indirectly help boost serotonin by enhancing the absorption into the brain of tryptophan, the amino acid that can be converted in the body to serotonin. However, eating very sweet, refined foods is not a long-term solution. Although they may give you temporary satisfaction, the speedy processing of such foods by the body leaves you craving more soon afterward. It is much better to eat unrefined, naturally high-fiber carbohydrates, such as an oat bar, wholegrain crackers with houmous, or fruit with yogurt. See page 70 for a list of foods that boost your serotonin levels and therefore help to prevent you from craving sweet, starchy foods when you are feeling low.

Balancing blood sugar

The main problem with bingeing on very sweet, refined carbohydrates is that they rapidly raise your blood-sugar levels. When your blood sugar drops again, so does your mood. (The role of blood sugar in balancing mood is explained in detail on pages 12–17.)

It is therefore essential to take measures to maintain even blood-sugar levels as part of a strategy to prevent uncontrollable urges to eat. Try to have small, regular meals. Eat a balanced breakfast made up of slow-energy releasing foods (see the chart on page 16) so that you are not tempted to binge as a result of a mid-morning slump in blood-sugar levels. Snack between meals on fruit and nuts or a natural, live yogurt. Limit your intake of sugar and sugary foods and refined, highly processed foods, which are also full of sugar, as these send your blood-sugar levels seesawing, as do stimulants. A diet of fresh, unprocessed foods will even out your blood-sugar levels and make you far less likely to overeat. The mineral chromium can help the mechanism which controls blood-sugar levels—take 100 mcg at breakfast and lunch.

Allergy or addiction?

Some people seem to crave foods to which they are intolerant, and in eating these foods become "addicted" to them. It is possible that the foods we are sensitive to leave us momentarily feeling better, less depressed, or less groggy by having an opiate-like effect. However, this "high" does not last, leaving us in another slump and craving more. By detecting and eliminating from your diet any foods that you may be addicted to (see pages 38–9 for details), you may well be able to control your food cravings and stop binge eating.

RECIPES TO HELP PREVENT BINGEING

BREAKFASTS: Very Berry Breaky (page 83); Poached Eggs with Asparagus (page 83; pictured)
LIGHT MEALS: baked potatoes with toppings (pages 86–7); Red Cabbage and Feta Salad (page 90)
MAIN MEALS: Trout with Sunflower Seeds (page104); Broiled Mackerel on a Bed of Stinging Nettles (page 105); Sesame Stir-Fry (page 106); Sweet Roast Lamb (page 109)
DESSERTS: Apricot Ice Cream with Pistachios (page 118); Cardamom Fruits (page 118); Tropical Whizz (page 122)

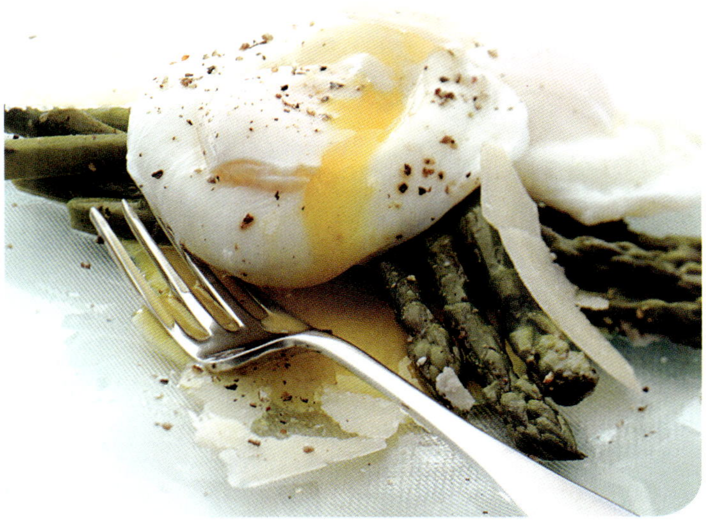

Your brain is the sun of your body's universe. From it radiates everything you do—every thought that crosses your mind, every memory you recall, every single movement you make. Whatever you are doing, you can count on your brain's help. Or can you?

brain slow-down

On the list below, tick the symptoms that are familiar and persistent for you:

- ☐ deteriorating memory
- ☐ finding it harder to do mental arithmetic
- ☐ people pointing out that you repeat yourself
- ☐ difficulty sustaining concentration
- ☐ easily confused by matters you used to take in your stride
- ☐ increasingly losing belongings

If you ticked three or more symptoms, you may be experiencing the effects of age-related cognitive decline, or ARCD. Thinking more slowly and poor memory recall are generally considered to be unavoidable features of ageing, and many of us notice them from our 30s onward. Of course, there are certain bodily functions that tend to change or deteriorate as we grow older, but these changes are not necessarily inevitable. By eating a balanced, healthy diet and taking appropriate nutritional and herbal supplements, you can keep ARCD to an absolute minimum. According to some scientists, you can even reverse it.

Healthy nerves

Your body's ability to maintain sharpness of mind and a good memory depends significantly on the health of your nerve cells. The efficiency at which messages travel along your nerves and through your brain is, in turn, largely dictated by the condition of your brain cells, or neurons, and their casing. Each neuron has a protective sheath around it called myelin, which is broken up at intervals. Messages literally bounce from one of these intervals to the next. When the message reaches the end of the neuron, it needs to be relayed across the tiny gap between the cells known as the synapse. To make this possible, chemicals called neurotransmitters are released from the first cell. These cross the gap and dock into the next cell, thus transporting the message across. In order to retain optimum brain function, you need to provide your body with the raw materials—a constant supply of proteins, enzymes, salts, and other molecules such as glucose and calcium ions—that it needs to produce healthy neurons and neurotransmitters. Essential fatty acids (see pages 26–9) play an important role in the health of brain cells. You can boost your intake of these fats by eating plenty of oil-rich fish, nuts, and seeds.

B vitamins are also important for sharpening mental acuity, particularly B6, B12, and folic acid, of which the

BITE-SIZE SOLUTION

To improve your brain function, try taking daily fish-oil supplements that are rich in omega-3 fats, particularly DHA (docosahexaenoic acid) and EPA (eicosapentaenoic acid). To protect these delicate fats from damage, include plenty of fresh fruit and vegetables in your diet to ensure an adequate intake of antioxidant nutrients (see page 130). If you are on medication, you should check with your doctor before taking food supplements.

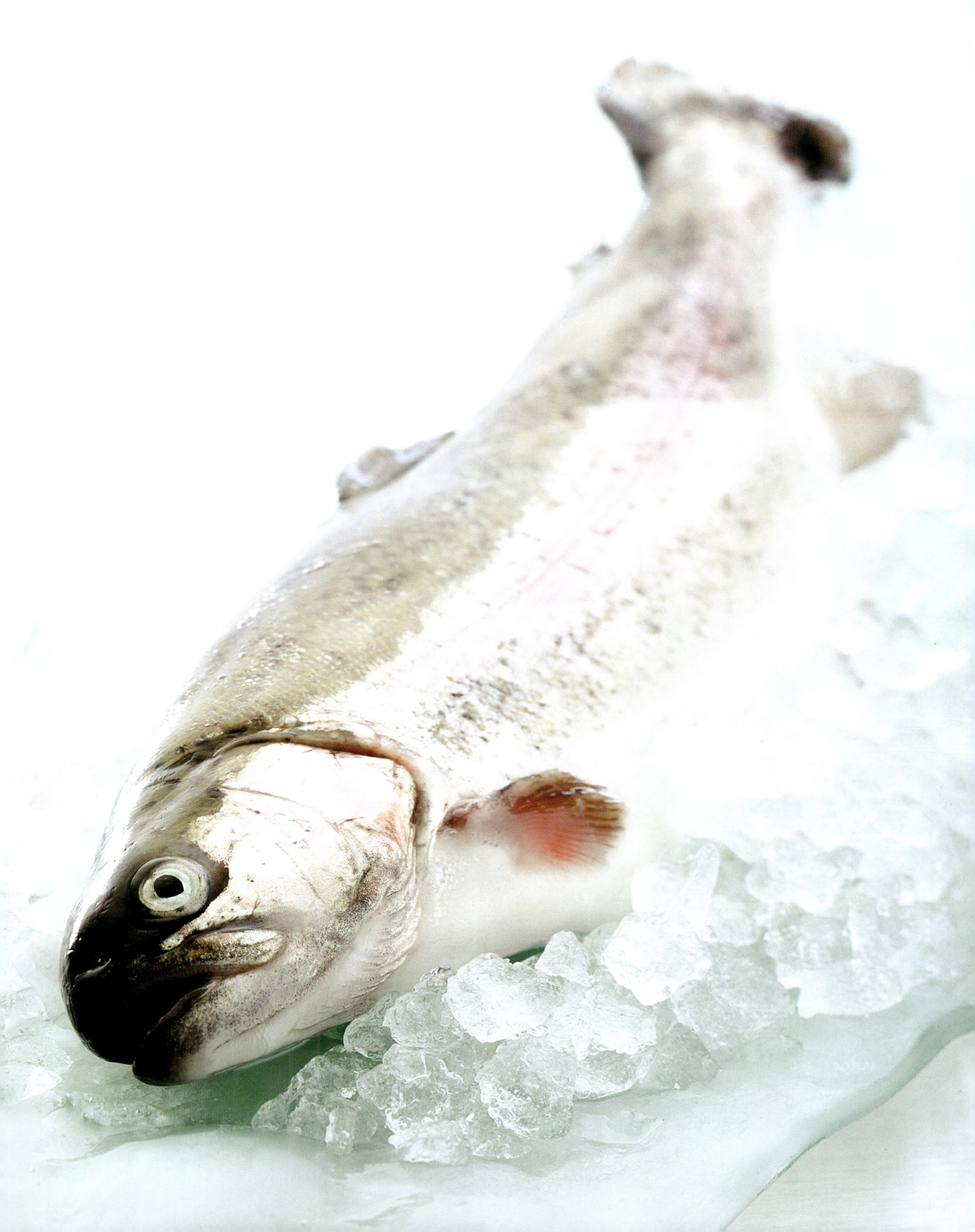

ACTIVE INGREDIENT: CHOLINE

Choline, which is a member of the B-vitamin family, has two major functions in the body associated with memory and the brain: It is needed for the structure of brain cells and also to make one of the key messaging neurotransmitters.

Provided there is a good supply of all the B vitamins and other nutrients, the body uses choline to produce phosphatidyl choline, which is incorporated into the membrane of each brain cell. Healthy membranes are, of course, vital if messages such as those that trigger memory are to be transmitted efficiently.

The transmission of memory messages also depends on the body's supply of acetylcholine, the main neurotransmitter responsible for memory and cognitive thinking. The body produces acetylcholine from choline. Some scientists have shown that a lack of choline can result in neurons cannibalizing their own membranes for the choline needed to make acetylcholine.

Although the human body can make small amounts of choline in the liver, this is usually not enough to maintain healthy brain cells, so we need a regular intake of choline through our diet. Many foods contain choline (or at least phosphatidyl choline). Particularly rich sources are cauliflower, eggs, fish, liver, milk, and legumes (such as peanuts and soybeans). A large egg is likely to contain 200–300 mg of choline. In a study of healthy elderly people, those given 500 mg of choline a day performed better on memory tests and reported fewer memory lapses than those not taking it. If you are eating a varied diet that includes some of the foods mentioned above, you are probably providing your body with the generally recommended intake of 500 mg a day.

Lecithin, which is a substance derived from eggs or soy, contains about 20 percent phosphatidyl choline and about 13 percent choline, although some brands are specially formulated to contain more. You can sprinkle lecithin powder on cereal or soups to increase your daily choline intake.

The following recipes are particularly rich in choline:

BREAKFASTS: Scrambled Eggs on Rye (page 80); Very Berry Breaky with soy yogurt (page 83)

LIGHT MEALS: Nanna's Rice Salad with eggs (page 88); Duck-liver and Artichoke Salad (page 91)

MAIN MEALS: Frittata (page 100); Fish Stew Provençale (page 102)

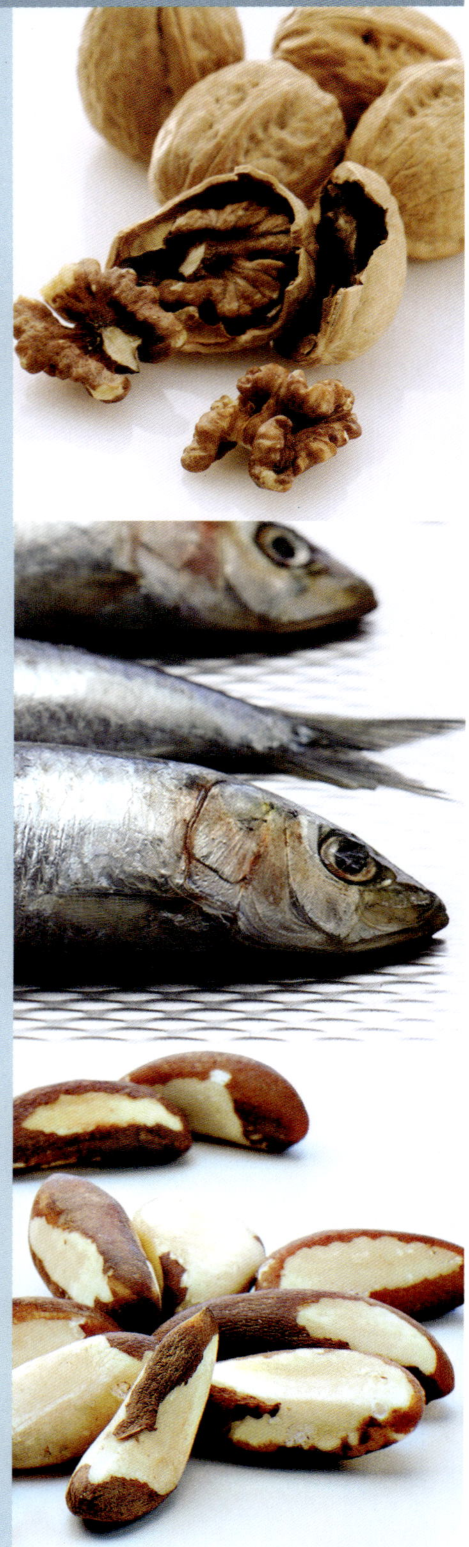

brain requires a constant supply. Good sources of B vitamins are whole grains, fish, lentils, most vegetables, wheatgerm, and sunflower seeds (see also box, page 46).

The B vitamins' role may be linked to the way in which they keep nerves healthy and help the production of substances called phospholipids—such as phosphatidyl choline (see box, opposite) and phosphatidyl serine—that combine with EFAs to make cell membranes.

Antioxidants

It is equally important to ensure that your nerves are well protected. The rich fat content in the neuron's protective myelin sheath and in cell membranes makes them particularly susceptible to attack by oxidants. These by-products of oxygen are like "sparks" and are produced by anything burning, including cigarettes, cooking fat, and petrol, and even by our own body's process of "burning" food to produce energy inside our body cells. Oxidant "sparks" damage cells, thereby making the body more vulnerable to disease and accelerating the ageing process, which includes a decline in nerve health. The body therefore needs a good supply of antioxidant nutrients, which protect it by acting rather like fire-proof gloves. In fact, researchers have found that people with higher blood levels of anti-oxidants tend to score better on memory tests.

Key antioxidants are vitamin E (contained in seeds, nuts, and wheatgerm), vitamin C (fruits and vegetables), vitamin A and beta-carotene (orange or red foods), glutathione (onions and garlic), anthocyanidins (berries and beets), and other more potent ones such as the oil from thyme. See the list of antioxidant-rich foods on page 130 for more details.

Air supply

A major cause of memory decline is a reduction in the oxygen supply to the brain. The brain uses up a massive 20 percent of the oxygen in our body at any given time and any reduction in this can have profound effects (the most extreme of which is a stroke, when part of the brain is completely starved of oxygen by a blockage in a blood vessel). As we age, many of us have a build up of plaque deposits in our blood vessels, not least the ones that supply the brain with blood, the carotid arteries. The build up of arterial plaque in the carotid arteries literally reduces the size of the gap in the artery, thereby allowing less blood—with its crucial supply of oxygen, glucose, and other nutrients—to reach the brain. Cardiovascular disease, the cause of arterial plaque build up, is one of the major modern illnesses. Yet leading a healthy lifestyle and eating a balanced diet that is rich in fruit, vegetables, whole grains, and fish, and low in fatty, processed foods, as described in chapter 3, can go a long way toward preventing cardiovascular disease.

RECIPES TO COMBAT ARCD

BREAKFASTS: Filling Fruit Bowl (page 80); Designer Muesli (page 83)

LIGHT MEALS: Creamy Tuna and Smooth Salmon baked-potato toppings (pages 86–7); Japanese-Style Tuna Salad (page 92);

MAIN MEALS: Kebabs (page 102); Broiled Swordfish in Caper Salsa (page 102); Broiled Rainbow Trout (page 104); Broiled Mackerel on a Bed of Stinging Nettles (page 105); Salmon Rolls (page 106); Thai-Style Icefish (page 106); Seatown Kedgeree (page 109)

DESSERTS: Baked Bananas with Raspberry Sauce (page 121); Crunchy Oaty Crumble (page 121; pictured below)

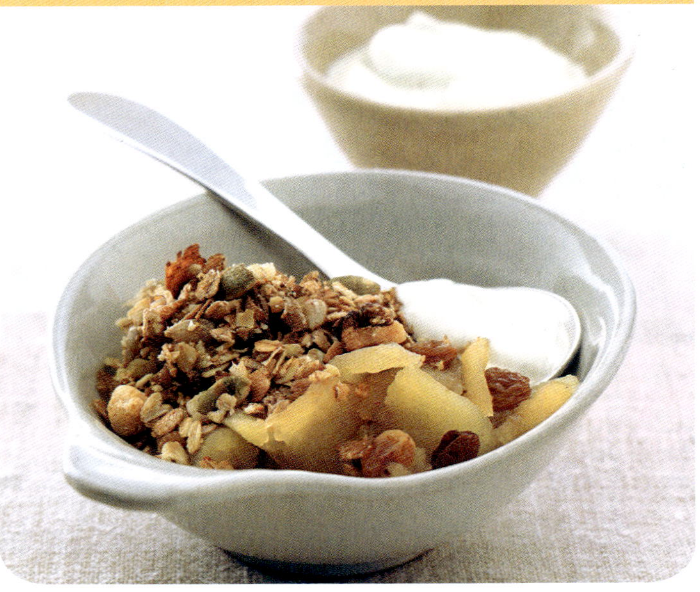

All too often, underlying imbalances in the body that can trigger or worsen depression are not taken into account when treating the condition. Here we explore dietary methods that can help you to overcome depression and take back control of your emotional wellbeing.

depression

On the list below, tick the symptoms that are familiar and persistent for you:

- ☐ low mood
- ☐ lack of motivation for and pleasure from usual activities and interests
- ☐ poor concentration
- ☐ difficulty making decisions
- ☐ disturbed appetite—either loss of or increased
- ☐ disturbed sleep—either sleeplessness or oversleeping, often unrefreshed by sleep
- ☐ tiredness
- ☐ decreased sexual energy (libido)
- ☐ feelings of worthlessness and hopelessness
- ☐ anxiety
- ☐ physical symptoms that do not respond to treatment, such as headaches, digestive disorders, and chronic pain

If you ticked five or more of the above symptoms you may be suffering from a degree of depression.

We have all felt low at some time or another. For example, it is absolutely normal to feel sad following a bereavement, the end of a relationship, the loss of a job, a disappointment, or a severe illness. However, for some people, this sense of sadness goes on for months on end and permeates every aspect of their lives, leaving them unable to truly enjoy anything they do. They even suffer from physical symptoms, such as fatigue, sleep problems, and a change in appetite. Sometimes the sadness does not even have an obvious trigger; it just comes from nowhere in particular and lingers.

IMPORTANT NOTE

If you are feeling seriously depressed and have thoughts of self-harm you should consult a doctor immediately.

Such a persistent mood disturbance may continue as mild depression for years, or may be so severe that the sufferer is barely able to cope with normal daily life. Some level of depression is thought to affect as much as one fifth of the adult population in North America and Europe.

Mood disorders are notoriously difficult to categorize and deal with, because they can be triggered by countless different sources. It is clear that the physical and psychological aspects of depression are closely linked. Major life events have an impact on our physical health, which in turn may affect our emotions, particularly in the long term. Therefore, any approach to redressing mood imbalances must take into account both the physical and psychological aspects. Although the scope of this book is

BITE-SIZE SOLUTION

Eat regular meals throughout the day and include some fiber- and protein-rich foods at each one, such as fresh fruit and yogurt for breakfast. This can help even out your moods by maintaining a more level blood-sugar balance (see pages 12–17).

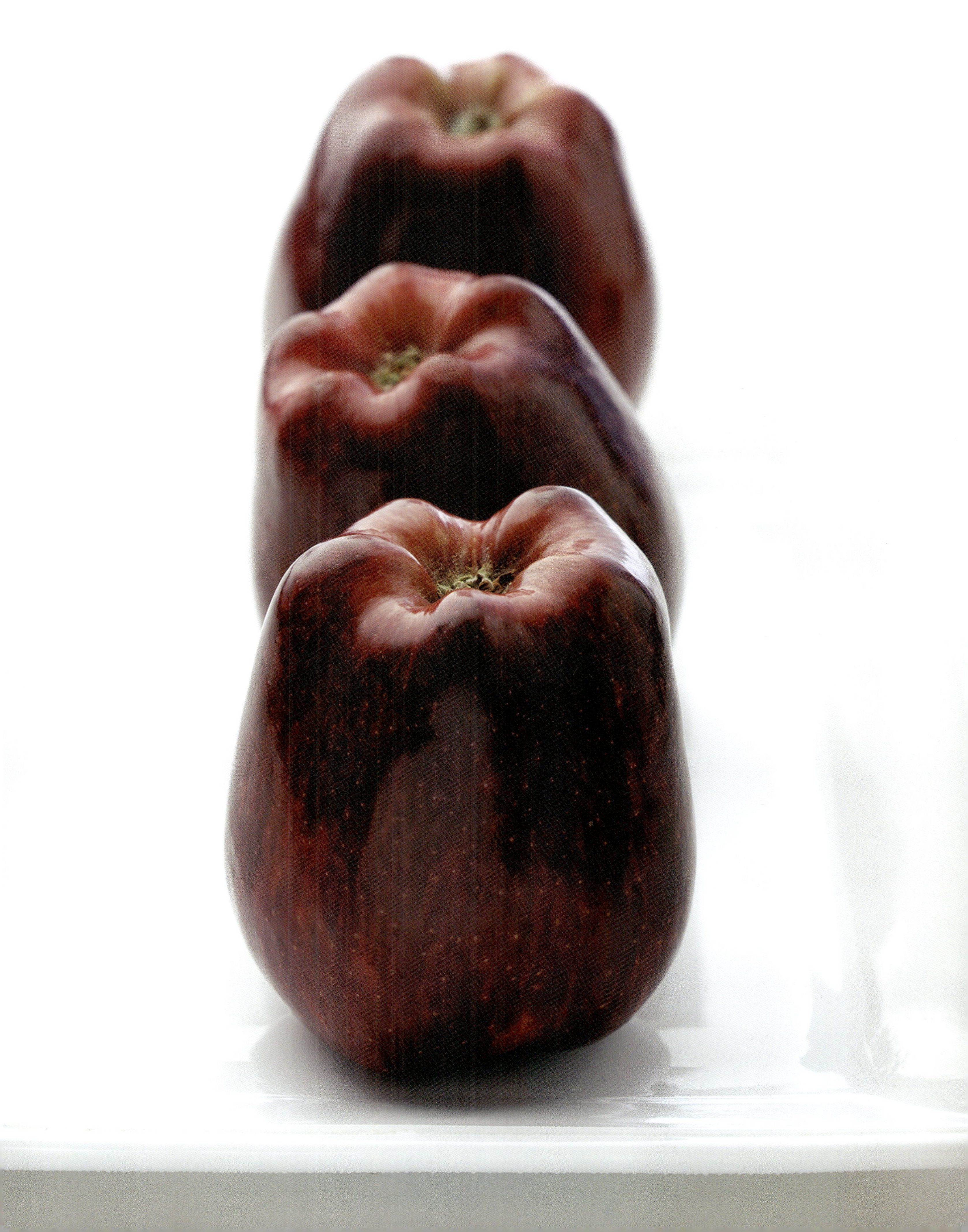

to focus on physiological strategies based on food, you will find advice on talking through problems on pages 134–5. Anyone suffering from severe depression should visit their doctor for a full medical evaluation of their condition. The information in this section is designed to help someone with mild depression—that is, persistently low moods—to identify and redress physiological imbalances that may be contributing to or exacerbating their condition. Ideally, except in the case of severe depression, such a strategy should be your first course of action. Unless these organic factors are dealt with, the success of any other treatment—be it drug or psychotherapy—will inevitably be compromised.

If you have been feeling low for a long time, there are several possible underlying imbalances that could be affecting your body. These are all covered in more detail in Chapter 1. In this section, we take a brief look at each type of imbalance specifically in relation to mild depression.

Nutrient deficiencies

Almost every process in your body relies, to a certain degree, on nutrients from your diet (see pages 22–5). A good intake of nutrients is particulary important in balancing moods. Nutrients are required to produce the brain chemicals needed for keeping your mood up, maintaining healthy brain and nerve cells, and supporting all the other body processes that can, if under par, lower your mood. Even a deficiency of a single nutrient can hamper the way your brain works. For example, research has shown low levels of vitamin B6 in people with depression—B6 is needed for the formation of serotonin and other neurotransmitters required to maintain good moods. In fact, all the B vitamins are important—low levels of vitamins in this group have been linked to a variety of behavioral changes, including depression, anxiety, irritability, and insomnia, among others. For a list of foods rich in B vitamins, see the chart on page 45.

In order to avoid nutrient deficiencies, alongside any other measures you are taking, you need to eat regular meals that are made up of nutritious, unprocessed foods. I also recommend taking multivitamin and B-complex supplements (or a high-strength multivitamin) in order to ensure that you are getting enough of every nutrient. (Do not take individual B-vitamin supplements without the guidance of a professional nutritionist.)

EXERCISE CAN MAKE YOU HAPPY

Regular, appropriate exercise may well be one of the most powerful antidepressants available. Many research studies have shown that low- or moderate-intensity physical activity can reduce levels of depression and anxiety, and that people who exercise on a regular basis feel better, have greater self-esteem, and are generally happier than those who do not. However, it is important to make sure you do not over do it, so start gently with a form of exercise that is not too strenuous, such as walking, swimming, or yoga. For more on the role of exercise in boosting your moods, see pages 132–3.

Essential fats

Fat is good for your brain, but not just any old fat. The omega-3 and omega-6 essential fats—found in oily fish, nuts, and seeds—are the best types of fat for fueling your brain and nerve cells (see pages 26–9). Essential fats, deficiencies of which have been linked to lowered moods, are used by the body to help fire messages more efficiently from one nerve cell to the next.

If you are feeling depressed, you will probably benefit from increasing your intake of the essential fats and cutting highly processed or animal fats from your diet. Medical research has shown that high levels of fats called triglycerides in the blood, often as a result of a diet high in animal fats, also affect mood. This is because triglycerides can cause blood to thicken, thus slowing the supply of oxygen to the brain. See pages 130–131 for a list of foods that are rich sources of essential fats.

Blood-sugar balance

One of the most crucial factors in balancing out your moods, concentration, and energy is maintaining even

STIMULANTS AND DEPRESSION

Several of the foods, drinks, and other substances we are likely to turn to when we are feeling down do stimulate our mood and energy. But the effect is never long-lasting or genuinely beneficial.

Alcohol puts a strain on your liver and irritates the lining of your digestive tract, making you more susceptible to gut problems and further liver overload. A high alcohol intake is also linked to depression for other reasons: A drinking binge causes blood-sugar levels to drop dramatically, taking with them your mood, energy, and concentration (see pages 12–17 for more on balancing blood-sugar levels, which can help if you find you crave alcoholic drinks). Alcohol also stimulates the release of the stress hormone cortisol, high levels of which have been linked to depression (see page 20). Drinking too much alcohol can disrupt your sleep too, leaving you feeling tired, irritable, and low.

Cigarettes can also play a part in depression. If you smoke, the nicotine in each cigarette kick-starts the body's stress mechanism in your adrenal glands (see page 18), which releases the hormone cortisol. In the long term, high levels of cortisol are linked to depression. Recreational drugs such as marijuana also fall into this category, so if you tend to get depressed you should avoid them.

Research has shown a greater incidence of depression among people with a high intake of coffee, another well-known stimulant. People are also more likely to drink coffee when they are depressed. Like nicotine, coffee stimulates the release of cortisol.

Sugar is another "quick-fix" substance that has a negative effect on mood (see main text, opposite and pages 12–17 for details on the role of blood sugar).

blood-sugar levels (see pages 12–17). When we are stressed, down, or upset, our body's ability to keep our blood-sugar levels relatively stable is impaired. At such times, we usually make things worse by not eating regularly and by turning to stimulants such as coffee, tea, cigarettes, sweet foods, and alcohol. All of these interfere with blood-sugar balance, creating a vicious cycle of ups and downs and eventually continual downs. Scientific studies have shown that people who are even mildly depressed have difficulty maintaining stable blood-sugar levels, so taking action to avoid dramatic fluctuations is essential.

Avoid sugary, processed foods and stimulants and increase your intake of foods and drinks that provide a more sustained solution. See page 13 for a list of foods that promote even blood-sugar levels.

Food sensitivities

Many people find that eliminating certain foods from their diet can have a remarkably beneficial effect on their mood. See page 39 for a list of foods that most commonly trigger mood changes, along with information on how to identify and eliminate such problem foods from your diet.

Hormone balance

Long-term stress has a dramatic effect on hormonal function, often causing mild depression. For a detailed look at whether you may be suffering from a hormonal imbalance owing to stress, see pages 18–21.

Once the body has reached the stage where stress is affecting hormonal balance, which in turn is triggering depression, there is no quick fix. It takes time to redress the balance by reducing your stress levels, learning better coping strategies and giving your body what it needs on the physiological front. This involves eating a nutritious diet aimed at maintaining even blood-sugar levels and taking supplements, such as vitamin C and B vitamins, that help to restore efficient functioning of the adrenal glands.

Toxic overload

When your body is overloaded—whether that is with too much food, foods that are not nutritious, excess alcohol,

ACTIVE INGREDIENT: TRYPTOPHAN

By eating foods that are rich in the amino acid (protein building block) tryptophan you can help raise your body's levels of the mood-boosting neurotransmitter serotonin (see page 20). Considerable quantities of tryptophan are found in the following foods: Chicken, bananas, figs, milk, tuna, turkey, seaweed, sunflower seeds, and yogurt. However, you need to be aware that eating large amounts of these foods (apart from being somewhat repetitive) is not a guaranteed way of making sure that the tryptophan they contain will actually be converted into serotonin in the brain.

For a start, tryptophan can also be transformed into other substances once it has been absorbed into your system. Secondly, you need a good supply of certain nutrients—such as vitamins B3, B6, C, and folic acid, biotin, and zinc—for the conversion into serotonin to take place. There is also another potential drawback: When you eat foods that contain other amino acids (that is most protein-rich foods), they tend to beat tryptophan to the transport vehicles that carry it across into the brain, leaving your serotonin raw material on the outside. However, eating foods rich in carbohydrates, even if they do not contain tryptophan themselves, helps increase the amount of tryptophan from other foods that is actually transported across into the brain, as there is less competition for the carriers. This is probably why many people crave starchy or sweet foods when they are feeling down—to raise serotonin levels.

To increase your levels of tryptophan, and thus serotonin, you should try to include some tryptophan-rich foods in your daily diet. Also, make sure you have some unrefined, wholesome, carbohydrate-rich foods (such as brown rice or wholegrain bread) with every meal, and generally follow a healthy, varied, balanced pattern of eating. Take a multivitamin/mineral supplement (see page 128) to ensure an intake of the whole spectrum of nutrients needed.

The following recipes are rich in tryptophan:

BREAKFASTS: Filling Fruit Bowl (page 80); Very Berry Breaky (page 83)

LIGHT MEALS: Mediterranean Chicken Salad (page 84); Open Spicy Tuna Sandwich (page 88)

MAIN MEALS: Trout with Sunflower Seeds (page 104); Gobble Pie (page 109); Shiitake Roast Chicken (page 110)

DESSERTS: Baked Bananas with Raspberry Sauce (page 121)

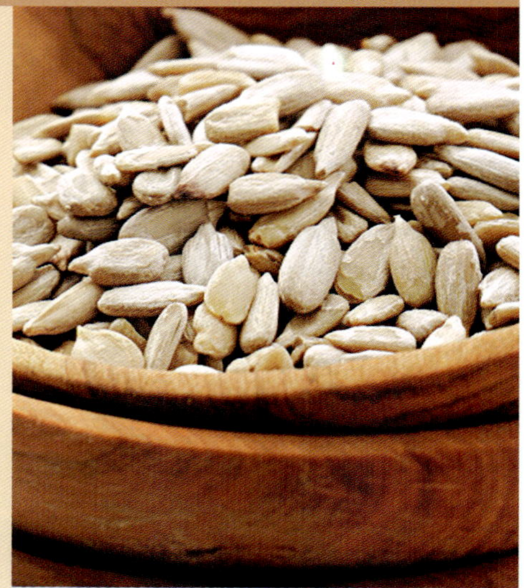

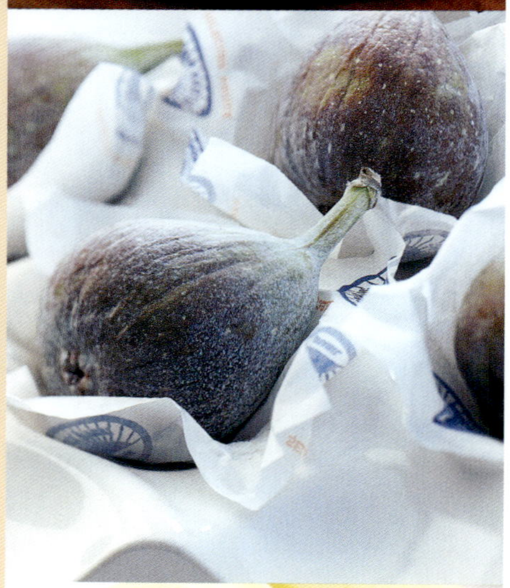

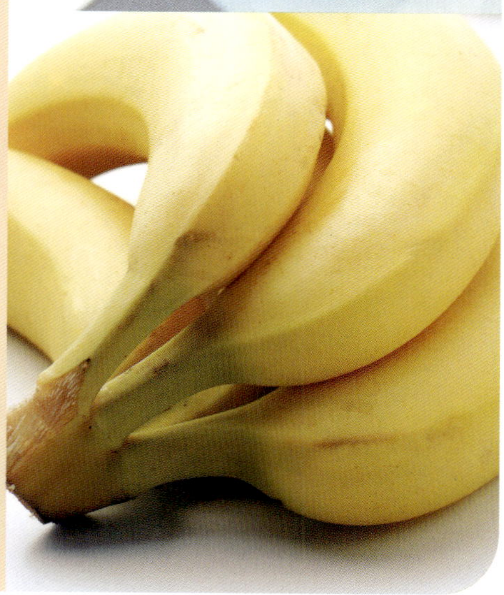

environmental toxins, or drugs (prescription or recreational)—you are unlikely to feel well either physically or emotionally (see pages 30–35). Toxins interfere with your brain and nervous system, in effect acting as neurotoxins. One adverse effect of some medication is depression, so if you are taking drugs and are depressed, you should talk to your doctor about this.

If you follow a gentle program aimed at enhancing your body's detoxification processes (such as the one on pages 36–7) you may well find your depression eases. You can also go a long way to reducing the burden on your system simply by eating a diet of fresh, unprocessed foods.

Mood chemicals

Modern psychiatry bases the treatment of mood problems on the manipulation of neurotransmitters—brain chemicals that act as messenger molecules, firing messages from one cell to the next. It is now well established that low levels of certain neurotransmitters are a key underlying cause of depression. Indeed, drug therapy involves medication that is designed to boost levels of certain important neurotransmitters such as serotonin and dopamine. Such drugs can be very effective and indeed life-saving if somebody is severely depressed. However, for many people suffering from mild depression who do not feel the need to resort to antidepressant medication, or who are reluctant to do so, there are several alternative, natural ways of raising your levels of mood-boosting neurotransmitters. For example, certain foods, including lean meat, dairy products, fish, and eggs, are known to help raise dopamine levels (see also page 53).

Ensuring that you have sufficient levels of serotonin in your brain is one of the most important natural methods of combating depression. See the box opposite for details on increasing your serotonin intake through your diet.

Diet for a mood boost

Any diet aimed at improving mood is pretty much the same as a diet aimed at maintaining all-round good health. There is no quick fix for boosting your mood with one particular food. Instead, you need to eat a wide variety of fresh, unprocessed foods that provide optimum nourishment and do not rob the body of nutrients, or overload it with sugar, saturated fats (such as those in animal products), salt, and food additives. So your diet is best made up of fresh fruit and vegetables, whole grains (for example, brown rice, oats), beans, seeds, nuts, some fish, lean meat, and low-fat dairy products. This way you will get the full spectrum of nutrients required to keep every system in your body functioning at its best, not least the mechanisms behind controlling moods.

As we have seen, following a diet that helps maintain even blood-sugar levels is crucial if you are trying to overcome depression. This means eating three regular meals a day, with snacks in between, of foods that are rich in their natural nutrients, fiber, and protein. Very sweet, starchy, refined foods should be avoided, as should stimulants such as coffee, tea, sodas, alcohol, and cigarettes.

On pages 10–39 you will find detailed dietary guidelines on how to balance the function of body systems and optimize your diet in order to maintain good moods.

RECIPES FOR LIFTING DEPRESSION

BREAKFASTS: Scrambled Eggs on Rye with Leeks and Mushrooms (page 80); Designer Muesli (page 83); Poached Eggs with Asparagus (page 83)

LIGHT MEALS: Baby Spinach and Goat's Cheese Salad (page 84); Smoked Fish Pâté (page 87); Japanese-Style Tuna Salad (page 92); Puy Lentil Salad (page 93); Fish Soup Provençale (page 97); Hot and Sour Soup (page 98)

MAIN MEALS: Fish Stew Provençale (page 102); Broiled Swordfish in Caper Salsa (page 102); Broiled Rainbow Trout (page 104); Broiled Mackerel on a Bed of Stinging Nettles (page 105); Salmon Rolls (page 106); Sesame Stir-Fry (page 106); Seatown Kedgeree (page 109); Barbequed Squid (page 110); Lentils with Spinach (page 110); Spiced Bean Stew (page 113)

DESSERTS: Apricot Ice Cream with Pistachios (page 118); Summer Whizz (page 122)

FAR FROM BEING MERE ESSENTIAL FUEL, FOOD CAN ALSO BE A SOURCE OF GREAT PLEASURE AND EMOTIONAL COMFORT. THE GUIDELINES PROVIDED IN THIS CHAPTER GIVE EQUAL EMPHASIS TO ALL THESE VALUABLE ASPECTS OF FOOD WITHOUT LOSING SIGHT OF THE IMPACT OUR DIETARY CHOICES CAN HAVE ON OUR HEALTH.

By eating fresh, healthy foods—such as the ones included in the diet and recipes described in this chapter—each day, you can dramatically improve your mood. It is important to ensure that every meal contains elements from each of the key food groups: Protein, because of its role in balancing blood-sugar levels; essential fats, which play a crucial part in brain messaging; whole grains and fiber-rich foods, which have a high nutrient content and help keep your system well-cleansed; and, of course, fresh fruit and vegetables, which provide an abundance of nutrients. And, as the inspiring recipes in this chapter show, "feel good food" can be truly delicious.

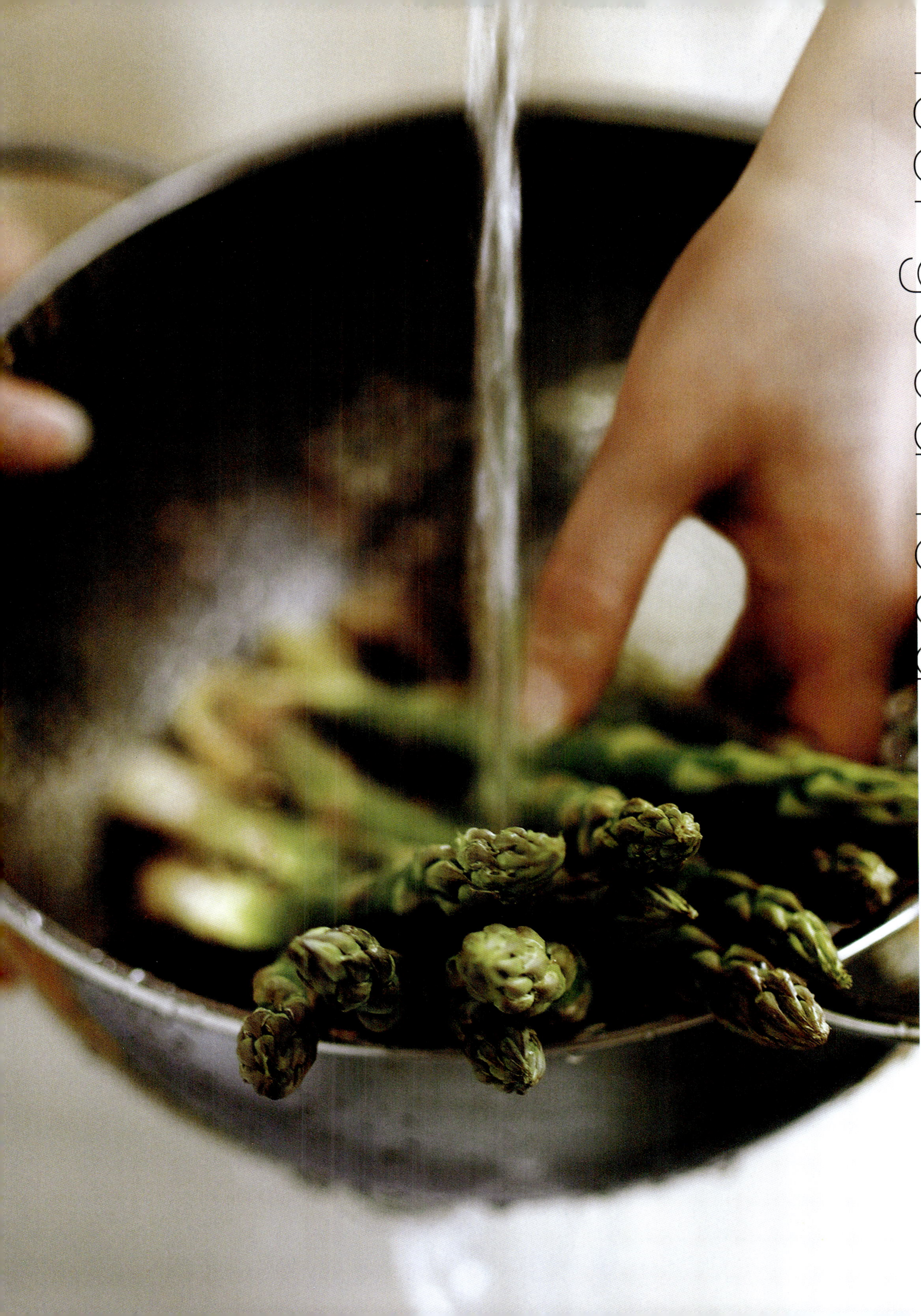

feel good food

Meals that help maintain good moods, generate high energy levels, and minimize illness are made up of fresh, unprocessed, varied ingredients put together in an appealing and inspiring way. In this chapter we outline the guiding principles of healthy eating and give a range of recipes.

feel good diet

Dietary strategies aimed at improving your mood—and, at the same time, optimizing all aspects of your physical and mental health—are outlined in detail in chapters 1 and 2 of this book. However, we do not always manage to translate these theories into the food on our plates: Busy lifestyles, bad dietary habits, and the apparent convenience of less healthy foods often take over. Yet by recognizing the powerful impact of eating good food and following some general strategies for boosting your moods and energy levels, it becomes remarkably easy to take the principles outlined in this book with you pretty much anywhere you go.

FEEL GOOD DIET BASICS

The basic qualities of any healthy, balanced diet are:

- freshness
- variety
- eating food as close to its natural state as possible
- pure water

These basics translate into practice like this:

- drink at least 3 pints (1½ litres) of pure water per day
- have fresh, colorful vegetables, raw, lightly steamed, or stir-fried twice a day
- have at least two pieces of fresh fruit daily
- eat plenty of fiber-rich foods, such as beans, lentils, whole grains, fruit, and vegetables
- eat a variety of lean proteins (including some vegetable protein, even if you are not vegetarian), such as eggs, lean meat, and poultry, beans, soy produce, dairy produce
- limit the amount of sugar you add to foods and drinks, and avoid it in sweetened foods
- limit your intake of refined foods (white bread, white rice, and so on), processed foods, and fast foods
- limit your intake of tea and coffee; good alternatives are herb/spice/fruit teas, or so-called coffee alternatives
- limit your intake of fatty and fried foods—broil, bake, poach, or steam instead
- limit your alcohol intake and avoid cigarettes

FEEL GOOD DIET PRINCIPLES

In addition to the basics, here is a reminder of the underlying dietary principles aimed at improving your overall mental wellbeing, described in chapter 1 of this book:

Balance your blood-sugar levels

- eat small meals five or six times a day, including fiber- and protein-rich foods in each one
- always eat breakfast
- dilute fruit or vegetable juices with 70 percent water
- eat fruit with protein, such as natural yogurt, a handful of nuts, cottage cheese, and so on
- avoid sugar, foods containing sugar, honey, and dried fruits
- avoid refined, processed foods
- avoid coffee, tea, alcohol, and cigarettes

Get adequate essential fats

- have cold-pressed unrefined seed oils on salads, stirred into soups, on oatmeal, or neat

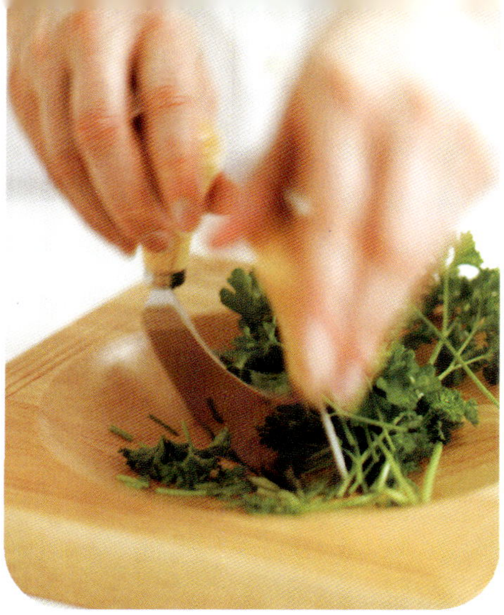
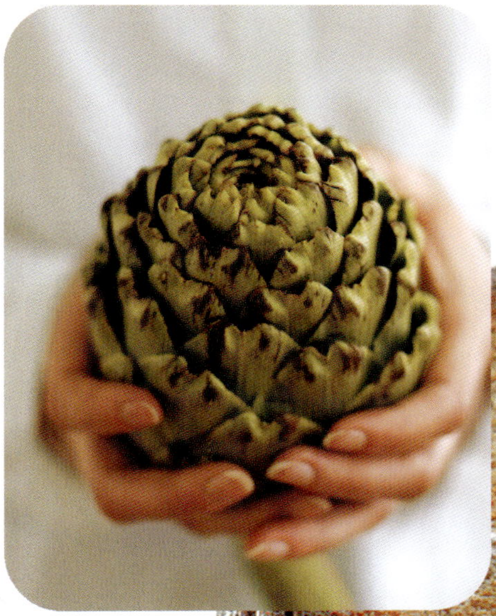
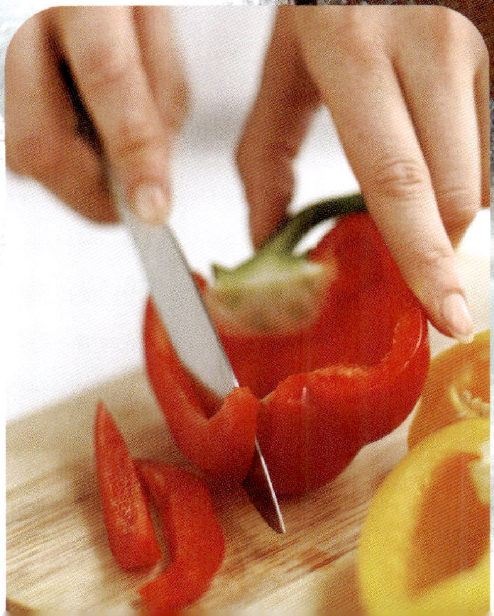
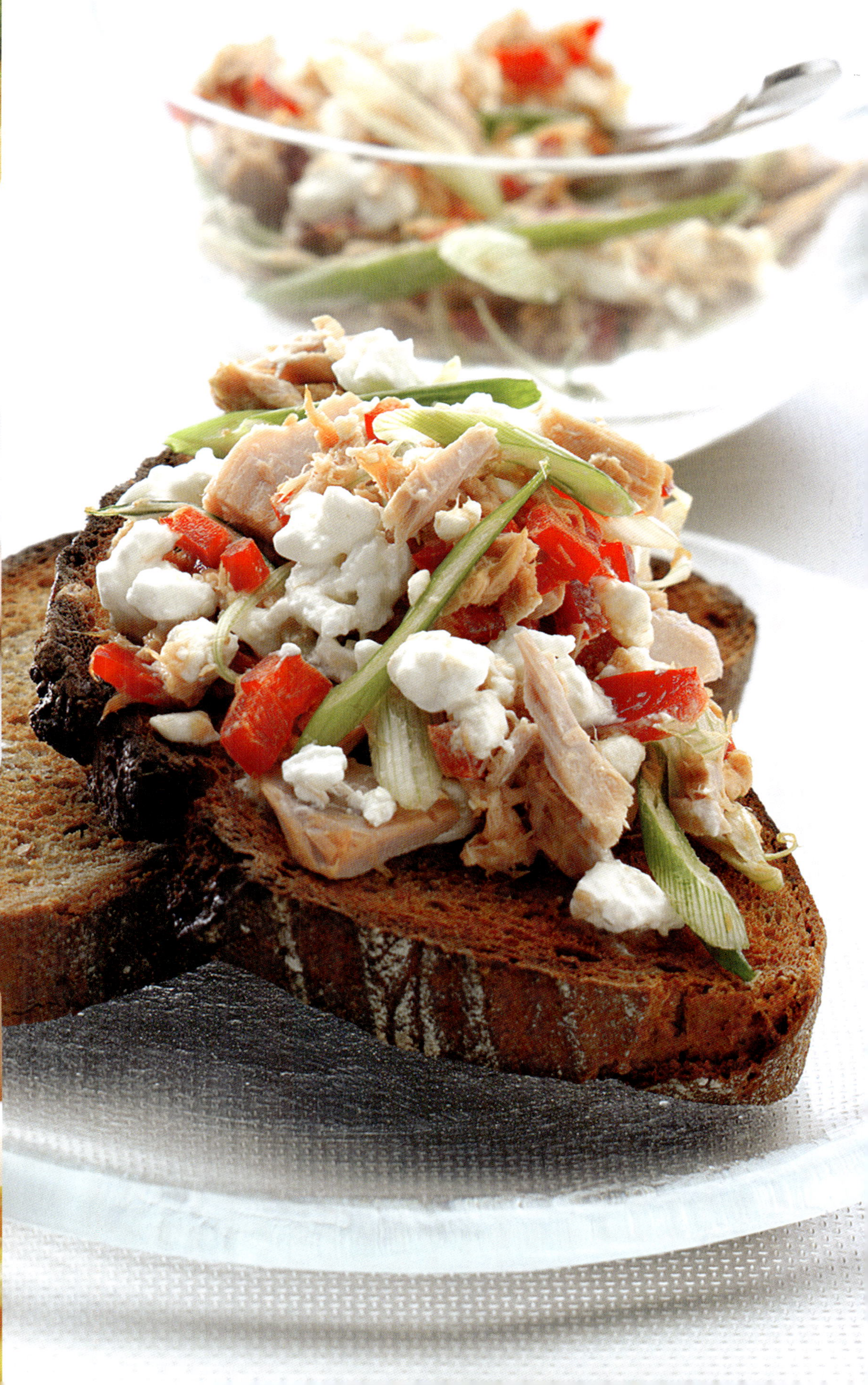

- grind a blend of pumpkin, sunflower, sesame, hemp, and flax seeds, and sprinkle on cereal, soup, and salads
- use whole pumpkin, sunflower, and sesame seeds on salads, as snacks, or on cereal
- have oil-rich fish, such as salmon, mackerel, sardines, tuna, or Antarctic icefish, at least three times a week
- use olive oil for cooking
- limit your intake of saturated fats from meat, dairy produce, and coconut milk
- avoid all refined, processed oils including processed foods containing them (look out for "hydrogenated fat" in the list of ingredients)
- avoid fried foods—broil, bake, poach, or steam instead
- eat plenty of fresh fruit and vegetables

Optimize your digestion and detoxification

- eat plenty of fiber-rich foods, such as beans, lentils, whole grains, fruit, and vegetables
- avoid refined carbohydrates, such as sugar, white bread, pasta, cakes, and so on
- avoid all processed, pre-packaged foods, and fast food
- avoid fried and fatty foods
- limit your intake of tea, coffee, and alcohol

Identify and eliminate food sensitivities

- assess which foods you eat daily and which you crave—common "offenders" are wheat, gluten, and dairy products
- see the full list of common triggers on page 39; follow the guidelines on how to test for and identify these
- eliminate allergens from your diet, choosing good alternatives (perhaps with the help of a healthcare practitioner) to ensure you are not missing out on important nutrients
- avoid foods you appear to be sensitive to, again, making sure your diet is not too restrictive

Maximize your nutrient intake

To maintain a balanced mood and even energy levels, you need to eat regular meals that contain "nutrient-dense" foods. In other words, foods that are giving you maximum nutrient value, without putting a strain on your body by demanding more nutrients for processing than they provide. It's therefore important to make sure you are getting a good

THE MAKE-UP OF A HEALTHY MEAL

This diagram represents the proportions of fresh vegetables, protein, and starch contained in an ideal meal for keeping blood-sugar levels as even as possible. While such a meal is digested and its nutrients are released to produce energy, dramatic fluctuations in blood-sugar levels are avoided.

Sticking to these proportions of fresh vegetables, protein, and starch most of the time will help you to maintain even moods and energy levels. However, bear in mind that the diagram represents an ideal, and need not be applied to every meal you eat. For example, some very healthy meals, such as fruit with yogurt for breakfast, may contain no starch at all. Simply use this diagram as a basic eating guide, to which you should regularly add essential fats and pure water.

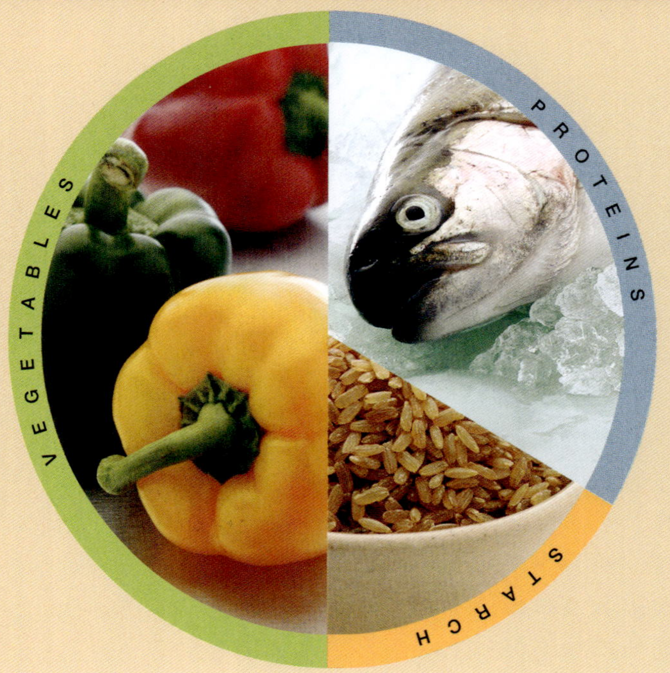

daily intake from the key food groups—protein, essential fats, whole grains, and fiber-rich foods, and, of course, fruit and vegetables, which provide an abundance of nutrients. The recipes on pages 80–125 have all been labeled with symbols to show which major nutrients they contain.

EATING OUT

Eating away from home—whether during the working day, business lunches, or going out for dinner—is increasingly common. It may seem like hard work to follow the principles of Feel Good Food when you do not have absolute control over your meals, but it can actually be very easy to do.

For example, breakfast at work or on the run could be a piece of fruit, a small pot of natural yogurt, and a handful of nuts or seeds. A good take-away lunch might be: A baked potato with a protein-rich filling (such as tuna, cottage cheese, or eggs) and a salad; sushi; rice salad; soup (keep your own rice, oat, or rye crackers at your desk to have with it); or a bag of raw, washed vegetables from the supermarket with cooked chicken, cottage cheese, or houmous.

If you are going out for a meal, my advice would be to just enjoy it: Choose whatever you fancy from the menu and make the most of the occasion. However, if you want to follow the recommendations in this book strictly, or you have to eat out regularly, here are some suggestions to bear in mind when selecting your meal:

- choose a light starter, such as rocket salad, broiled vegetables, or a non-creamy soup
- go for a simple main course or ask for it to be cooked plainly, for example, griddled swordfish or baked chicken without a rich sauce
- order plenty of fresh, lightly cooked vegetables or a large salad to go with your main dish; explain that you would like to have more of these vegetabes than potatoes or rice
- if you order a dessert, share it with someone or just choose a fruit salad
- order a peppermint tea instead of coffee—this will not only help your digestion but also refresh your palate
- start with a large glass of mineral water, then alternate drinking a glass of wine with a glass of water, or drink spritzer (white wine with soda water)

FEEL GOOD RECIPES

The recipes on pages 80–125 are mostly influenced by my own experience. They feature flavors I remember from my early years in the Middle East, where I was born, and are also marked by the culinary cultures of my parents' birthplaces—Britain and the Mediterranean island of Malta. The Indian influence in our household during my childhood played an important part in molding my taste, too, as did the time I spent living in East Asia. Of course, years of nutrition training and working with countless clients have also shaped the underlying tone of the food I recommend. I aim to combine healthy eating with flavor and practicality. I am grateful to the many friends who have also contributed their favorite recipes, allowing me to spread the net of influences even wider.

The recipes here are all relatively straightforward to prepare, and involve minimum mixing, measuring, and washing up. Although the ingredients have been carefully listed and measured, most of the recipes are just as good when doctored to suit your own particular taste—do not be afraid to experiment with flavors and other ingredients. Each dish should be a creative experience to be savored; it should nourish the soul as well as the mind and body.

Symbols used to describe the recipes

Protein-rich food, such as eggs, yogurt, fish, tofu, or meat, helps make the meal more sustaining for your energy and mood.

Essential fats are just that—an essential part of our diet. They are particularly important for keeping nerve and brain cells healthy so that they can fire their messages appropriately.

Whole grains are naturally high in fiber and their full package of nutrients, just as nature intended. Fiber is also important for keeping your body's elimination and detoxification processes in good working order, making you less likely to feel sluggish.

Fruit and vegetables, nature's nectar, provide us with a huge range of healing and protective nutrients as well as fiber and water.

(Servings are approximate.)

pantry

Most of us could probably do our regular supermarket shopping blindfolded, with the same items gracing our basket each week. If you are a seasoned visitor to the "wellbeing" aisle or healthfood stores, you are likely to be familiar with most of the suggestions below. If you are not, you are about to discover a new world of wonderful flavors to use in your kitchen. Either way, one of my main shopping mottos is to vary the contents of my basket from week to week, trying to stick as far as possible to local produce that is in season—this is the next-best thing to growing your own food. I'm also someone who (mistakenly) feels there's no food in the house if the fruit bowl and the vegetable drawer in the refrigerator are empty, no matter how packed the cupboards are with dried or canned foods. Actually, you can make some delicious, healthy meals—such as the Spiced Bean Stew on page 113—with not much more than a few cupboard staples plus an onion.

Washing fruit and vegetables

Always wash all your fresh fruits and vegetables thoroughly, even—or perhaps especially—the organic ones. When I get home from the shops, I fill the sink with water, add a few crystals of potassium permanganate (available at any pharmacist) and a capful of vinegar, and put all the fruit and vegetables in to soak. Rinse well. Some, such as leeks and strawberries, are best washed just before you use them, rather than before you store them in the refrigerator.

Organic

Ideally, buy as much organic produce as you can afford and is available. That way you minimize your toxin intake, perhaps getting more nutrients (although the jury is still out on that one), supporting a more sustainable environment, and helping bring the cost of organic food down. Don't be fooled, though, into thinking that if something is organic it is, de facto, good for you. An organic cookie, or organic coffee made with organic cream and sugar, is still high in sugar, flour, caffeine, and saturated fat.

Rice

The best rice to use is brown basmati; not only does it have a fantastic flavor and texture, but it also provides plenty of fiber and is a slower-releasing rice than any others. I have an automatic rice cooker (available at Asian shops), which takes all the work out of getting the water-to-rice ratio right. A great way to add flavor to a meal is to cook the rice in stock instead of plain water. You can pop in a few cloves of garlic for extra flavor. A teaspoon of turmeric will turn the rice yellow and give it an extra antioxidant boost.

Tamari

This is a type of soy sauce. It is made without wheat and is available at most healthfood stores. Check out the Japanese section of healthfood stores for other flavorings and condiments.

Seaweed

There are several types of dried Japanese seaweed available, which you can add to soups, or rehydrate and include in salads. Seaweed has a subtle, yet distinctive flavor and provides you with a wealth of important minerals. Some brands make excellent condiments, such as black and white sesame seeds mixed with seaweed in a bottle—a quick topping for any dish.

Oils

I recommend using a good quality, extra-virgin olive oil for most recipes. Most healthfood stores sell delicious, cold-pressed seed oils such as sunflower or pumpkin. Otherwise, there are a couple of excellent blends of high-quality, essential fatty acid-rich oils available, which you can buy through your nutritionist. I'd recommend experimenting with all of these oils on salads, or poured over dishes once they've been cooked.

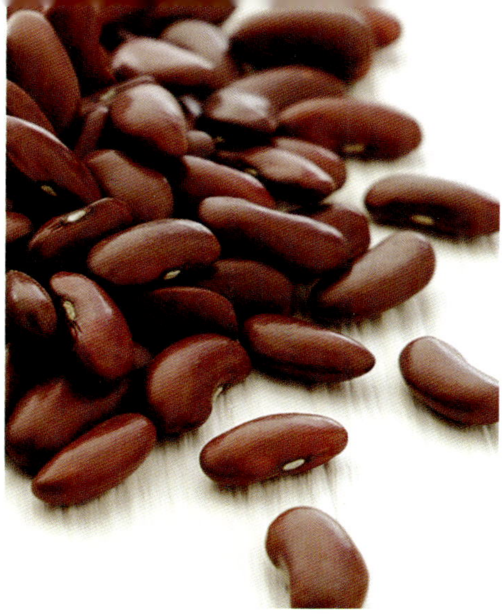

Never use cold-pressed seed oils for cooking as heat damages them.

Salt

Anyone who has high blood pressure or problems with water retention is generally better off avoiding salt. Of course, salt does enhance the flavor of a meal—if you really can't resist using it, just try to do so sparingly. Get into the habit of tasting your food first, and then adding a little salt if necessary. Seasalt is a good choice—I'm a great fan of a blend of seasalt and herbs. It is also possible to buy special salt that is naturally low in sodium and relatively high in the important mineral potassium.

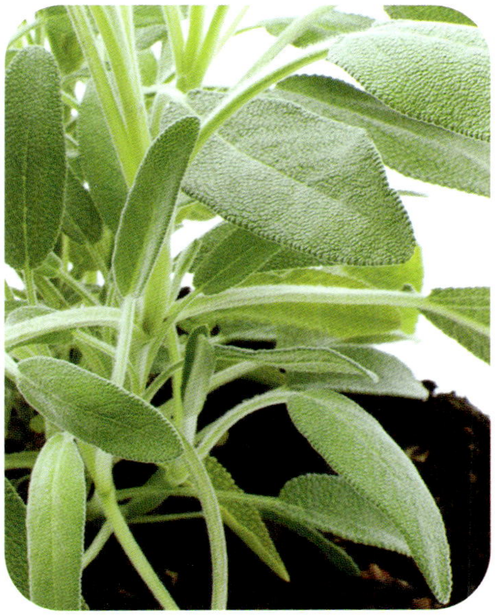

Herbs

Fresh herbs can make a huge difference to a dish. If you're not used to cooking with them, experiment with flavors. Herbs that are particularly good raw in salads are fresh basil, coriander, and parsley, while thyme is my favorite for cooking. Note the difference between fresh coriander and ground coriander—the latter is a spice, a powder of coriander seeds whose flavor bears no resemblance to the fresh, green leaves so popular in Eastern Asian dishes.

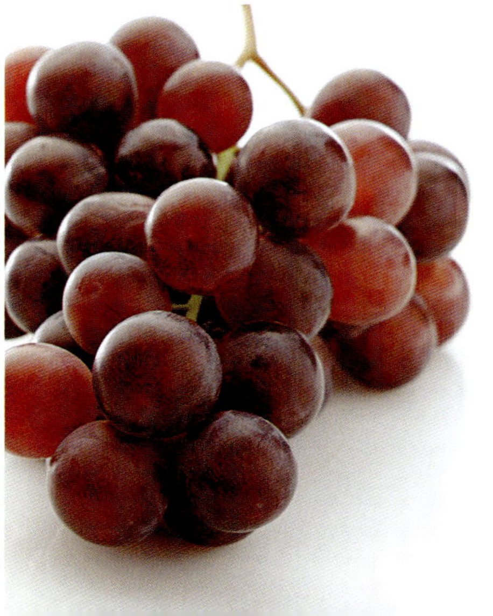

Seeds

There is a recipe for the High-Five Seeds mix on page 82. Because it contains hemp and flaxseeds, this is best ground up. However, pumpkin, sunflower, and sesame seeds are great tossed into salads and other dishes. These seeds are particularly tasty toasted, although the fat content is damaged in the process, so aim to use them raw most of the time. To toast seeds, lay them on a tray in the oven until they start to brown. Alternatively, toss them continuously in a large skillet (with no oil) until they start to turn brown, but keep a close eye on the seeds—they turn very quickly from tasty brown to burnt.

Drinks

You can't beat pure water as far as drinks go, so make sure you have at least 2–3 pt (1–1½ l) a day, although if you eat plenty of fruit and vegetables you are probably fine on a little less. I recommend mineral or highly filtered water. For other drinks, check your healthfood store for a wide range of herb and spice teas. Experiment, as there are so many, you may be surprised to find a few you really like. My favorites are spice-blend teas—there are some truly wonderful ones available—or standards like peppermint and chamomile. There are several "coffee alternatives" made from dandelion root, endive, and so on. In my view, these don't come close to the real thing, but may provide a good alternative if you are cutting down on the hard stuff. Steer clear of sodas (even sugar-free), fruit cordials, and sweetened juices—go for fresh, pure juices and dilute them with some water. Smoothies made with yogurt or milk are a filling snack drink, but the pure fruit ones can raise your blood sugar too quickly.

breakfasts

The notion of enjoying a breakfast fit for a king and reducing the size of your meals as the day goes on until you are eating like a pauper for dinner is a wise one. Eating well in the morning kick-starts your metabolism and sets you up for the day. It also replenishes your fuel supplies after the night's fast, hence the name of the meal ("break-fast").

Some people really don't feel like eating first thing in the morning. There's nothing wrong with letting your body wake up for a while and having breakfast an hour or two after you get up, especially if you have to make an early start and would rather snatch a few more minutes in bed.

At breakfast it's important to have some protein, such as yogurt, soy yogurt, or eggs. This makes the meal satisfying and prevents your blood-sugar levels from plummeting soon afterward (see pages 12–17). Breakfast is also the ideal meal at which to have a good serving of slow-releasing carbohydrates, such as oats or wholegrain rye toast, to provide you with fuel for the day ahead.

FILLING FRUIT BOWL

(main image, opposite)

Choose your favorite fruits for this great start to the day. Ripe fruits give the most taste. If you select dried fruits, it is best to soak them in water over night. As they are very concentrated in sugar, just use a few dried fruits mixed with fresh.

8 tablespoons low-fat, natural yogurt, or soy yogurt
4–6 pieces or servings of fruit from the following list: banana, pineapple (canned in juice in winter), pear, apple sauce, berries (frozen or canned in juice in winter), apricots, peaches, nectarines, dried fruit
2 tablespoons ground High-Five Seeds (see page 82)

Put the yogurt into two bowls and pile the fruit on top, chopped into small pieces if necessary. Top with a heaped tablespoon of ground High-Five Seeds.
Serves 2

SCRAMBLED EGGS ON RYE WITH LEEKS AND MUSHROOMS

Creamy, soft eggs on rich rye toast with a side serving of leeks and mushrooms is one of my favorite weekend breakfasts, eaten leisurely, poring over the papers. For a richer, more decadent version, serve it with a couple of slices of smoked salmon topped with fresh dill.

1 large leek
8 chestnut mushrooms
4 organic eggs
dash of milk or soy milk
freshly ground black pepper
pinch of salt
1 teaspoon olive oil
1 tablespoon chopped parsley (optional)
1 teaspoon butter
2 slices wholegrain rye bread

Trim and slice the leeks and wash them well in a sieve. Wipe the mushrooms clean and slice them.

Beat the eggs in a bowl with a dash of milk or soy milk, freshly ground black pepper, and a pinch of salt, ideally a seasalt and herbs blend.

Heat the olive oil in a large saucepan and, on a low heat, start to cook the leeks and mushrooms.

Some people don't like parsley and eggs, but if this combination appeals to you, add freshly chopped parsley to the leeks and mushrooms just before you've finished cooking to give the meal a green freshness.

When the leeks and mushrooms are done, serve them on two plates. Put the bread in the toaster and quickly heat the butter in the pan.

Add the eggs and stir constantly on a very low heat until they are the texture you like.

Butter the toast lightly, put it on the plates next to the leeks and mushrooms and top with the eggs.
Serves 2

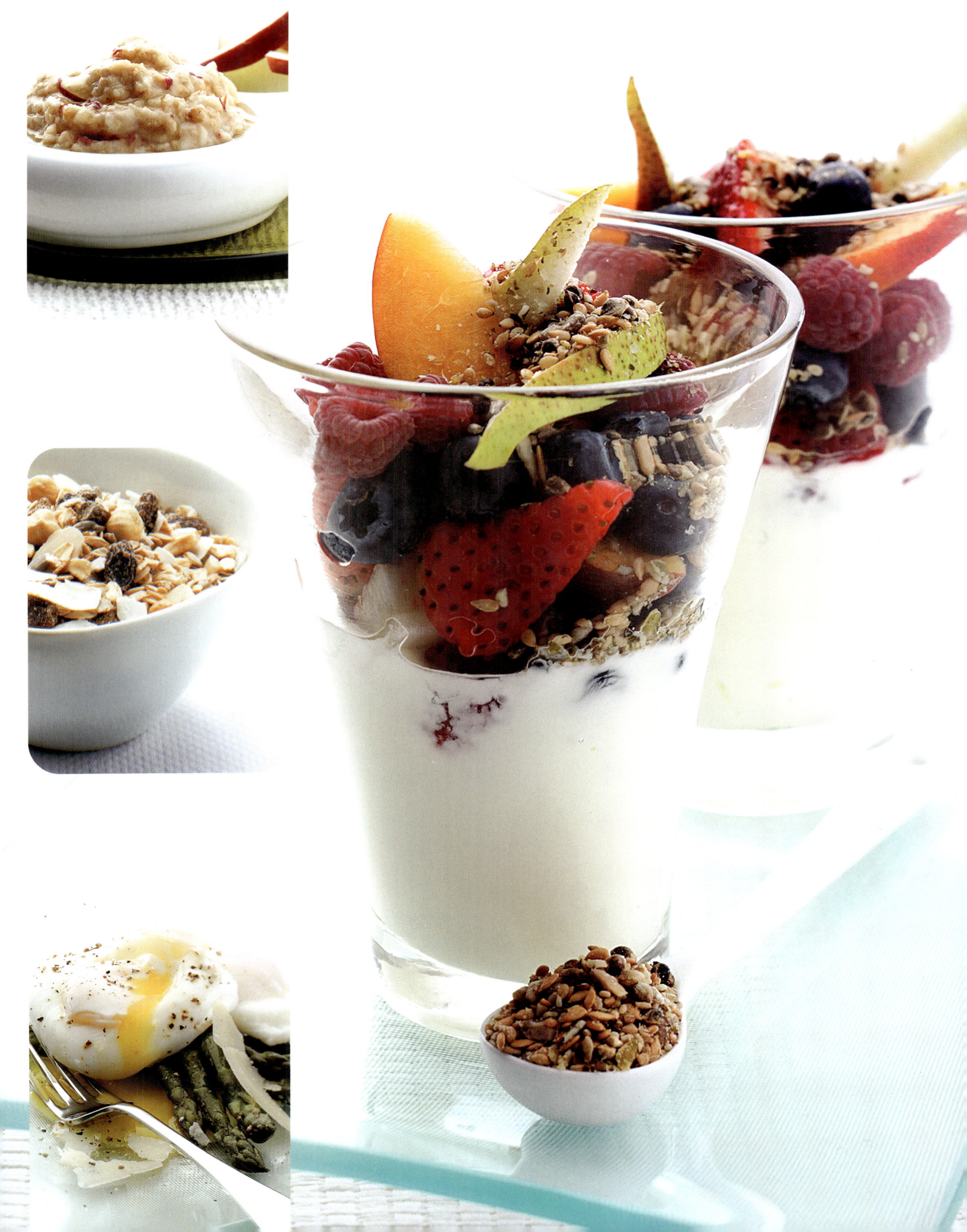

APPLE OATMEAL *(below)*

A great start to a winter's day. The apple adds an unusual texture.

5 heaped tablespoons oatmeal oats
some milk or soy milk to taste
1 apple, grated
1 teaspoon honey
½ tablespoon ground High-Five Seeds (see right)

Put the oats into a saucepan, cover with cold water, and stir gently over a low heat. As the oats begin to absorb the water, slowly add small amounts of milk, stirring all the time until the oatmeal is the consistency you like. When the oats are cooked—this should take about five minutes—stir in the grated apple and honey, sprinkle the seeds over the top, and serve immediately. Serves 2

HIGH-FIVE SEEDS

This blend of seeds, once ground up, can be used as a healthy, nutty topping for yogurt, cereal, soups, and casseroles. The seeds provide you with a good daily intake of the essential fats, as well as minerals—all in a tasty, versatile form.

You will need to mix together roughly equal amounts of the following seeds, all of which are available at healthfood stores: flax, pumpkin, sunflower, sesame, and hemp. These seeds are best eaten well ground. You could use a herb or coffee grinder (kept solely for that purpose of course, as you will no longer be able to use it for coffee beans). As the seeds contain a high percentage of volatile fats, which are easily damaged by heat and light, it is important to store the mixture in a sealable, airtight jar in the refrigerator.

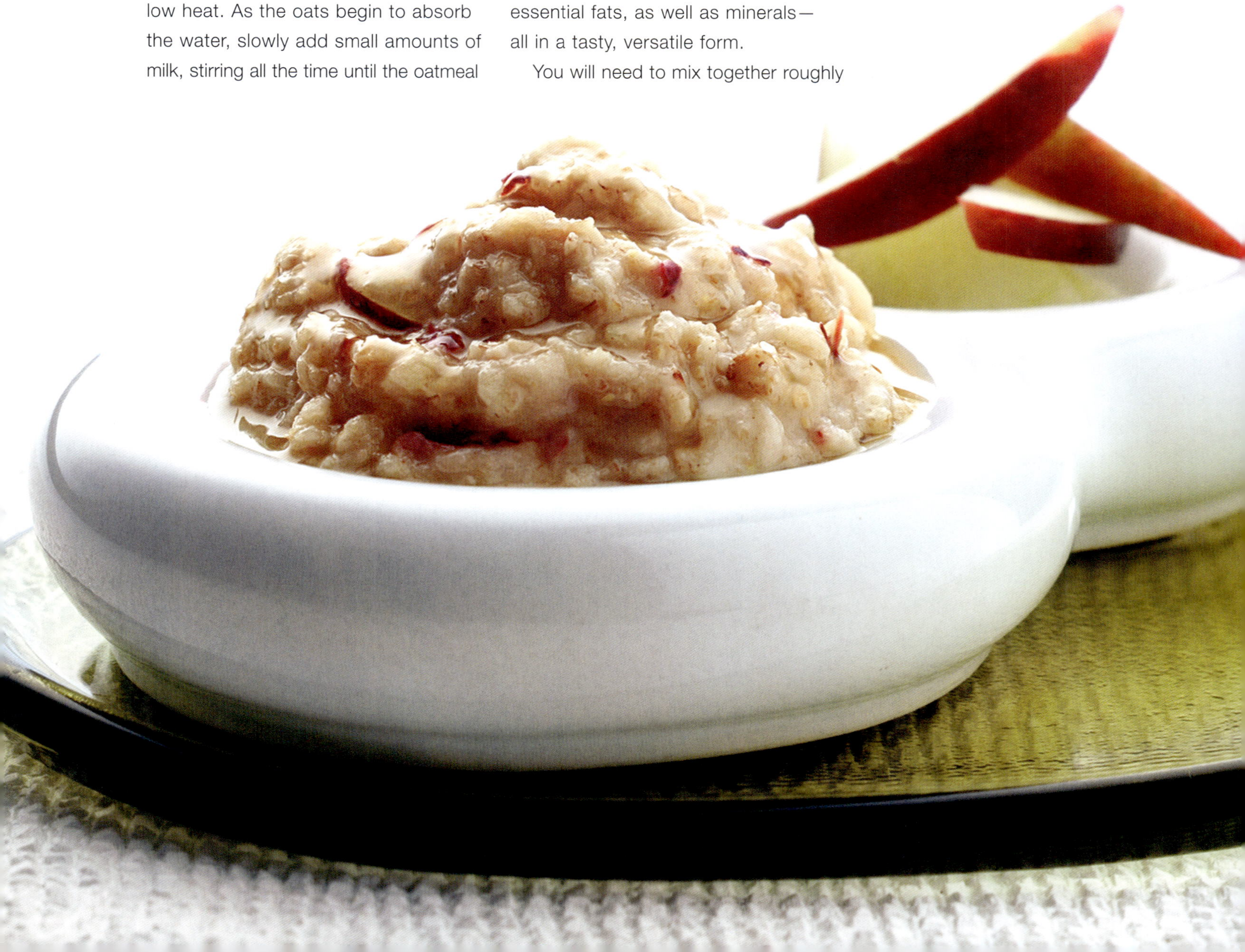

VERY BERRY BREAKY

Although this delightful smoothie is best made in the summer, using fresh berries—all that delicious taste and wonderful color—it's also good in the winter with frozen or canned fruit such as blackcurrants (canned in juice, rather than syrup).

6 tablespoons mixed berries, such as blueberries, strawberries, raspberries, blackcurrants, blackberries
8 tablespoons live, natural yogurt or soy yogurt
2 tablespoons wheatgerm
1 tablespoon essential-fat oil blend

Put all the ingredients in a blender for 1 minute and drink immediately.
Serves 2

DESIGNER MUESLI *(center inset image, page 81)*

This home-made muesli takes seconds to prepare, all to your own specifications. If you have a sensitive digestive system, you may find this easier to digest if you leave your bowl of muesli to soak overnight in milk or apple juice.

2 cups (200 g) oat flakes
2 cups (200 g) barley flakes
2 cups (200 g) rye flakes
2 tablespoons wheatgerm
1 tablespoon sunflower seeds
1 tablespoon pumpkin seeds
1½ tablespoons raisins or sultanas
8 dried apricots, finely chopped

Mix all the ingredients together in a large storage container with a lid. You can add any other nuts, seeds, or dried fruits you like. Good healthfood stores also sell a range of other grains (some are best puffed, such as quinoa, as they are inedible raw) that you can add to the mixture. Store in a cool place.

Have a bowlful of this muesli in the morning with fresh or soy milk or natural yogurt.

BUCKWHEAT CREPES

This is a variation on traditional French *galettes de sarrasin*—deliciously light pancakes. You can serve them with pretty much anything you fancy. I particularly like them with natural yogurt and blueberries or apple compote, or with a savory breakfast of scrambled eggs, vegetarian sausages, and baked beans. You could also try the crêpes with wilted spinach and crumbled goat's cheese.

¾ cup (100 g) buckwheat flour
pinch of salt
⅔ cup (150 ml) milk or soy milk
⅔ cup (150 ml) water
1 egg
olive oil

Put the flour and salt in a mixing bowl and add the egg. Mix the milk and water together in a jug. Beat the egg into the flour, adding the milk and water a little at a time to make a batter. Leave for at least 1 hour. Lightly oil a skillet and heat it well. Put a tablespoon of batter into the pan and roll it around to the edges. Cook it until the pancake is golden, then turn over to cook the other side. Serve hot with your choice of topping.
Serves 2

POACHED EGGS WITH ASPARAGUS *(bottom inset image, page 81)*

This is a wonderful—and rather sophisticated—breakfast or brunch dish. Scrambled eggs also go very well with asparagus.

20 asparagus spears
4 eggs
large knob of butter
Parmesan cheese
freshly ground black pepper

Trim the asparagus spears and steam them until they are tender right through, without allowing them to become too soggy. Meanwhile bring a pan of water to the boil. To poach the eggs, crack each one into a cup and gently slide it into the water, then stir the water quickly to create a whirlpool around the egg. After 3–4 minutes, remove the egg with a slotted spoon. (Alternatively, crack the egg into a ladle and hold it in the boiling water.) Place the asparagus in bundles on two plates and dot with butter.

Lay two of the poached eggs on each asparagus bundle and shave a little Parmesan over the top before sprinkling with black pepper. Serve with hot, buttered rye toast.
Serves 2

starters and lunches

These recipes are ideal as starters, or as a light evening or a lunchtime meal. Most of them take the barest minimum of preparation time, and some are great made in advance as a packed lunch. As with all the recipes in this chapter, experiment to suit your taste. For example, if you are vegetarian, have a couple of hard-cooked eggs instead of the chicken with the Mediterranean Chicken Salad (see right), or tofu with the Warm Chicken and Noodle Salad (see far right). If you don't like spicy food, leave the Tobasco out of the Spicy Bean Salad on page 89.

BABY SPINACH AND GOAT'S CHEESE SALAD

Baby spinach offsets a good-quality goat's cheese perfectly. (You can use feta cheese if you don't like the flavor of goat's cheese.) And with the High-Five Seed topping, you're getting a good dose of essential fatty acids, too.

½ lb (250 g) washed baby-spinach leaves
5 oz (150 g) fresh goat's cheese
1½ tablespoons ground High-Five Seeds (see page 82)
3 tablespoons Creamy or Tangy Vinaigrette (see page 114)

In a large salad bowl, toss the spinach with crumbled goat's cheese and vinaigrette and sprinkle with the seeds.
Serves 2

MEDITERRANEAN CHICKEN SALAD *(main image, opposite)*

This is one of my favorite quick lunches, and it couldn't be any simpler to prepare.

2 large handfuls of washed baby spinach
a handful of shredded red cabbage
4 scallions, finely chopped
8 cherry tomatoes, quartered
2 cold broiled or roasted chicken breasts

For the dressing:
1 tablespoon extra-virgin olive oil
4 basil leaves, torn or chopped
1 teaspoon coarse-grain mustard
2 teaspoons balsamic vinegar
freshly ground black pepper

Arrange half of the salad ingredients—spinach, cabbage, scallions, and tomatoes—on each plate and place the chicken breasts on top. You can use ready-roasted chicken from the supermarket if you are in a hurry.

Put the dressing ingredients in a jar and shake well. Pour the dressing over the chicken.

For an oriental spin, use the Oriental Bite Dressing, or, for a delicious French twist, the Tangy Vinaigrette (see page 114).
Serves 2

WARM CHICKEN AND NOODLE SALAD

You could replace the chicken in this salad with shrimps or tofu.

7 oz (200 g) rice noodles
4 baby corns
½ red onion
1 carrot
2 tablespoons shredded white cabbage
1 handful snow peas
1 tablespoon olive oil
1 clove garlic
¾ lb (350 g) chicken breast, skinned and boned
2 teaspoons sesame oil
2 teaspoons tamari or soy sauce
juice of 2 limes
1 handful fresh coriander, chopped

Cook the noodles according to the packet instructions. Drain, rinse in cold water, and place in a serving bowl. Wash, peel, and slice the vegetables. Crush the garlic. Slice the chicken into bite-sized pieces. Heat a wok or large pan and add the garlic and a tablespoon of water. Add the vegetables when the garlic is soft (not brown). Toss the vegetables until wilted. Add them to the noodles. Cook the chicken in the wok, stirring until it is cooked through. Add the chicken to the noodles. Toss together with the lime juice, sesame oil, tamari or soy sauce, and fresh coriander.
Serves 2

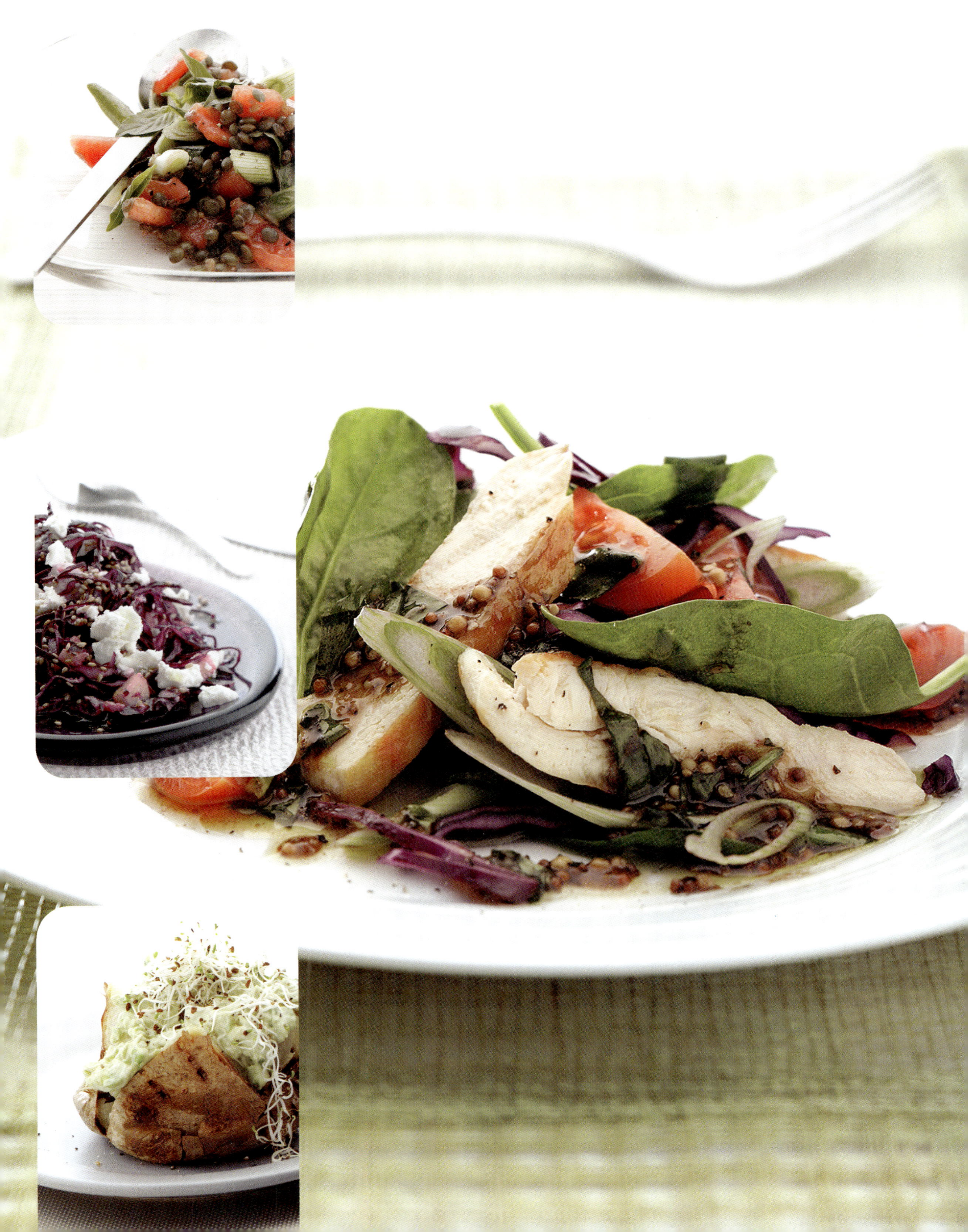

BAKED-POTATO TOPPINGS

A baked potato makes a filling lunch or quick supper. To cook your own potatoes, heat the oven to 350°F/gas mark 4, wash and prick the potatoes, and put them in the oven on a baking tray for about an hour, depending on the size of the potato. Check whether they are cooked through and soft by pricking them with a skewer.

If you buy one of those very large baked potatoes from a snack bar, it's best to scoop out some of the inside flesh. Otherwise you're likely to end up with a very big, starchy meal that may well send you to sleep later. Complement your baked potato with a Proper Green Salad (see page 114). Each topping serves 2

Houmous, Avocado, and Alfafa Topping *(below, left)*

4 tablespoons houmous
½ ripe avocado
2 handfuls alfalfa sprouts

Mash the houmous (bought ready-made from the supermarket) with the avocado and top with a handful of alfalfa sprouts.

Spicy Shrimp Topping *(below, right)*

5 oz (150 g) fresh shrimps
1 tablespoon natural yogurt
1 teaspoon tomato ketchup
dash of Tobasco sauce
squeeze of lemon juice

Boil the shrimps for 3–4 minutes until they turn pink. Do not overcook them, or they become tough. (You can use ready-cooked shrimps instead.)

When the shrimps have cooled, mix them in a bowl with the yogurt, ketchup, and Tobasco sauce. Add a squeeze of lemon and stir well.

Mustard Chicken Topping

2 cooked chicken breasts
2 tablespoons natural yogurt
1 teaspoon coarse-grain mustard
freshly ground black pepper
sprouted rocket and/or cress shoots

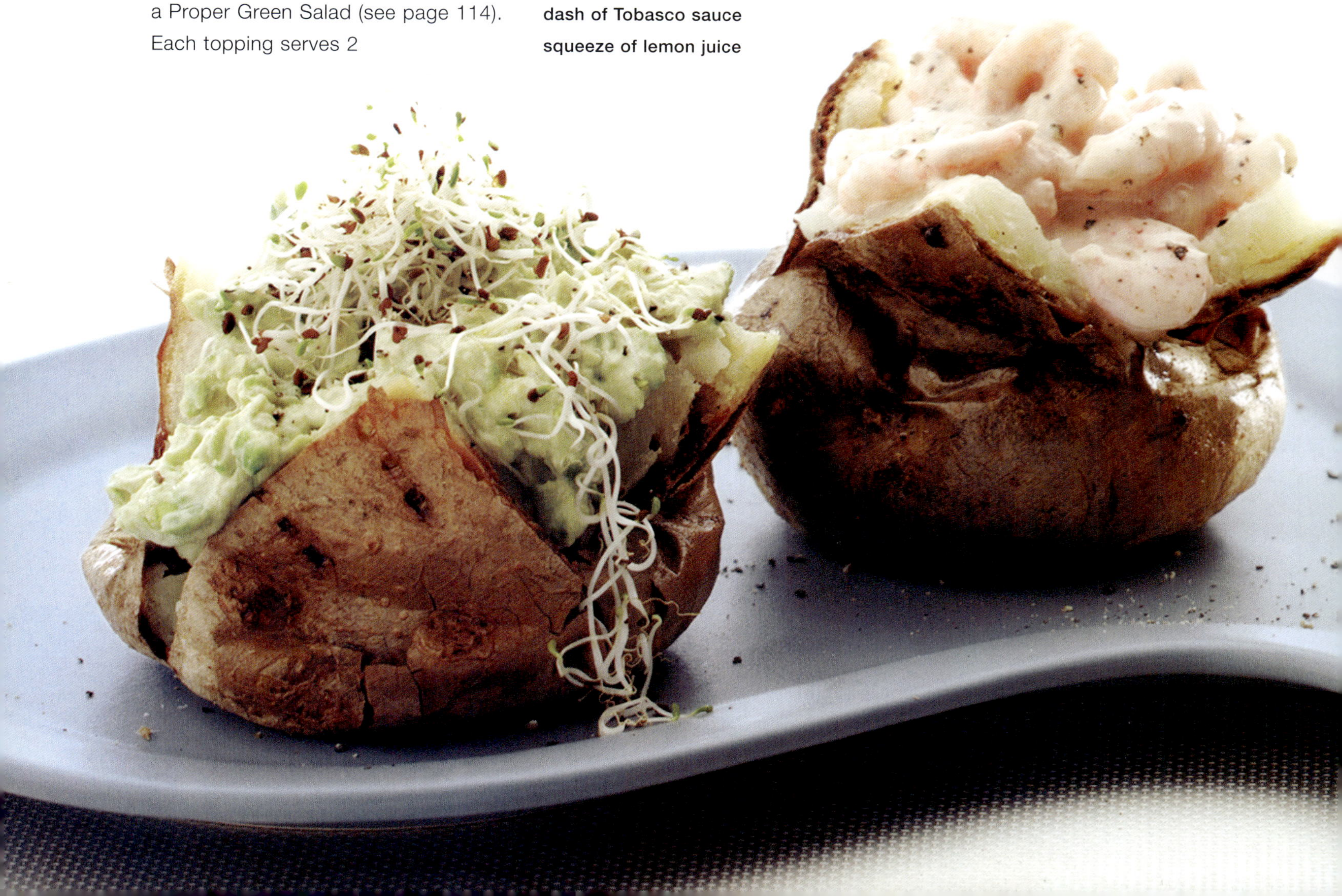

Dice the cooked chicken and mix it in a bowl with the yogurt, mustard, and black pepper. Top with the rocket and/or cress shoots, which are available at most supermarkets.

Creamy Tuna Topping *(below)*

1 7-oz (200-g) can tuna in brine
1 ripe avocado
½ red pepper, finely sliced
juice of ½ lemon
freshly ground black pepper
pinch of salt

With a fork, mash the drained tuna in a bowl with the avocado and the other ingredients.

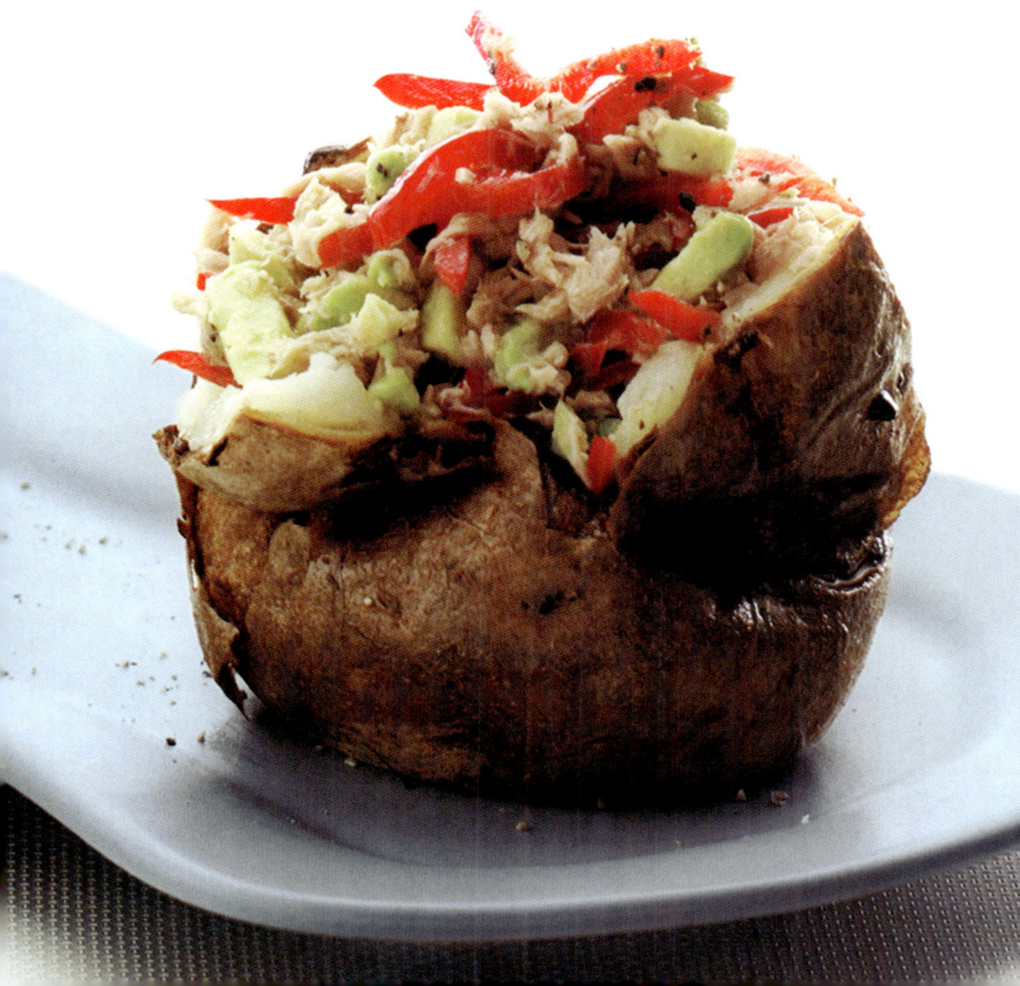

Smooth Salmon Topping

1 7-oz (200-g) can pink salmon
1 tablespoon cottage cheese
1 scallion, finely sliced
1 tablespoon chopped parsley
squeeze of lemon juice
freshly ground black pepper

With a fork, mash the drained salmon with the cottage cheese and other ingredients in a bowl.

SMOKED FISH PÂTÉ

This is an amazingly quick, easy dish to make as a starter or for lunch. To save time, I sometimes make it using ready-cooked mackerel fillets and mush it all up with a fork in a bowl.

2 oz (50 g) smoked haddock fillet
2 oz (50 g) smoked mackerel fillet
2 scallions
½ cup (110 g) cottage cheese
3 tablespoons water
2 teaspoons freshly squeezed lemon juice
1 tablespoon chopped parsley
a few slices of lemon
a few sprigs of parsley

Remove the skin from the haddock and poach in water for 15 minutes, or until it is cooked. Chop the scallions. Break both the cooked haddock and smoked mackerel fillet up into a blender and add the other ingredients. Put into a bowl and chill in the refrigerator until serving. Garnish with slices of lemon and sprigs of parsley. Eat with rye or rice crackers as a starter or with a large salad as a meal in itself.
Serves 2

CHICKEN AND MUSHROOM PÂTÉ

This is good for serving as a starter at a dinner party. It also makes a simple, satisfying lunch. You can vary the herbs to suit your taste.

4 medium-sized chestnut mushrooms
2 scallions
1 cooked chicken breast
4 tablespoons (50 g) cottage cheese
2 tablespoons olive oil
1 teaspoon chopped tarragon
1 teaspoon chopped parsley
freshly ground pepper
a pinch of salt

continued

Wash and trim the mushrooms, chop the scallions, shred the chicken and put them all in a blender with the other ingredients. For a rougher pâté, simply chop the chicken, mushrooms, and scallion very finely and mix all the ingredients in a bowl.

Put in the refrigerator to chill. If the pâté is for a dinner party, you can put it in four individual ramekin dishes.

Before serving, garnish with sprigs of fresh parsley or tarragon. Eat with rye or rice crackers as a starter or with a large salad as a meal in itself.
Serves 2 as lunch, or 4 as a starter

NANNA'S RICE SALAD

(opposite)

When I was a small child, my grandmother used to make a huge container of this for us to take down to the beach in Malta. This salad makes an excellent packed lunch. If you're not a fan of capers, you can use *jardinière*-style pickled vegetables, which provide a crunchy texture. I personally don't like putting eggs in, but they are part of grandmother Lizzie's original recipe. If you are vegetarian, try making the salad with just eggs, or replace the fish with cubes of smoked tofu.

1 cup (200 g) brown rice
3 eggs
3 large tomatoes
1 green pepper
4 scallions
12 olives
8 mint leaves
1 7-oz (200-g) can tuna in brine
1 heaped tablespoon capers
3 tablespoons olive oil
juice of ½ a lemon
freshly ground black pepper
pinch of salt

Cook the rice and set aside to cool. Boil the eggs until they are hard cooked and leave to cool.

Prepare the vegetables—peel, deseed, and roughly chop the tomatoes; finely chop the green pepper; finely slice the scallions; pit and chop the olives, and chop the mint. Add the drained tuna and all the other ingredients except the tomatoes to the cooled rice and toss the whole mixture well. Add the tomatoes just before eating. If you don't think you're going to eat all the salad in one sitting, just add tomatoes to individual plates, as they are likely to "turn" before the rest of the ingredients do.
Serves 2–3

OPEN SPICY TUNA SANDWICH *(main image, page 75)*

This sandwich gives a tasty touch to a can of tuna, and because it's "open" it automatically keeps your starch intake down.

7-oz (200-g) can tuna in brine
1½ tablespoons cottage cheese
½ red pepper, finely diced
1 red onion, sliced
½ teaspoon soy sauce
1 teaspoon olive oil
dashes Tobasco sauce
2 slices rye bread, toasted

Mix the drained tuna, cottage cheese, red pepper, red onion, soy sauce, and olive oil. Season with Tobasco to your taste—probably 2 or 3 dashes, but test in between in case it's too hot for you. Pile half the mixture on top of each slice of warm rye toast. This is great eaten alongside a Proper Green Salad (see page 114).
Serves 2

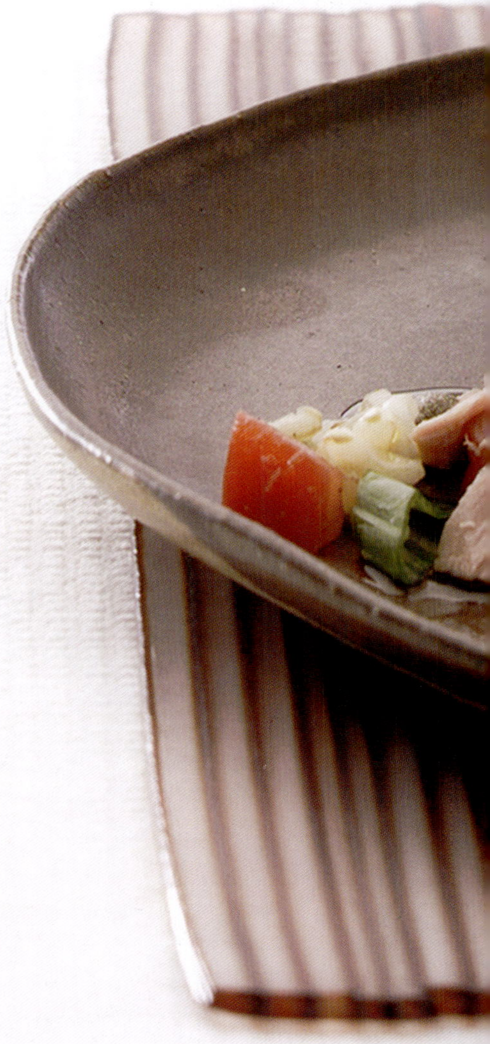

SPICY BEAN SALAD

This is a delicious and satisfying lunch, which takes no time at all to prepare. It's one of my staples when I'm working hard, and also makes a very portable packed lunch. Again, you can vary the meal's flavors by using one of the dressings that are described on page 114.

1 lb (420-g) can beans, such as pinto or mixed
1 large tomato, roughly chopped
2 scallions, sliced
10 scarlet runner beans, sliced
1 teaspoon soy sauce
2 teaspoons olive oil
1 tablespoon fresh coriander, finely chopped
dash Tobasco sauce

Mix the drained and rinsed beans with all the other ingredients and serve.

You can use parsley instead of coriander, and freshly ground black pepper instead of Tobasco. Or, for a more Mediterranean version, use lots of olive oil, lemon juice, and parsley with a bit of sea salt, leaving out the soy sauce, coriander, and Tobasco.
Serves 2

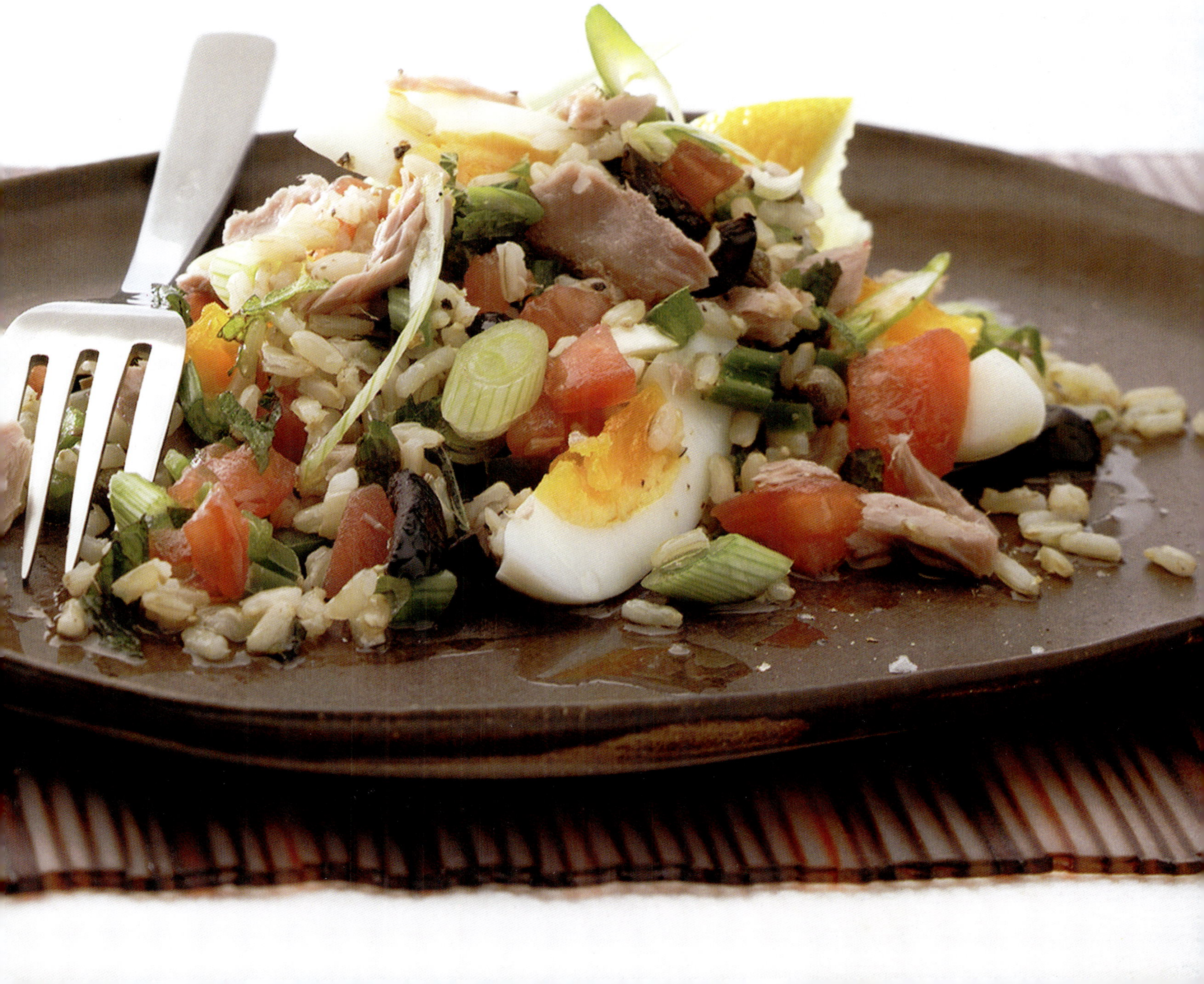

RED CABBAGE AND FETA SALAD *(below)*

The sharp taste and crunchy texture of red cabbage go beautifully with a rich feta cheese. Some people like to add a diced apple to this dish—this gives another texture, and the sweetness of the apple blends well with the other flavors.

½ large red cabbage
1 cup (150 g) feta cheese
1 apple, diced (optional)
2 tablespoons sunflower seeds
4 tablespoons Tangy Vinaigrette (see page 114)

Shred the cabbage very finely and mix with the crumbled cheese, chopped apple if you're using it, and sunflower seeds. Toss well in the vinaigrette.
Serves 2

DAHL

This is a slightly altered version of a traditional recipe that was given to me by Maria Pereira from Goa, who introduced my young taste buds to the aromatic flavors of Indian cooking. Dahl simply means "lentils," so it's just one of probably dozens of recipes using this Indian staple. This dahl is very quick and easy to prepare and freezes well.

1 cup orange split lentils
1 onion, chopped
5 cloves garlic
1 teaspoon olive oil
1 teaspoon ground coriander
1 teaspoon ground cumin
1 teaspoon ground turmeric
3 cups water
1½ cups (400 g) canned chopped tomatoes

Wash the lentils thoroughly in a sieve and remove any little stones. In a large saucepan, soften the onions and garlic

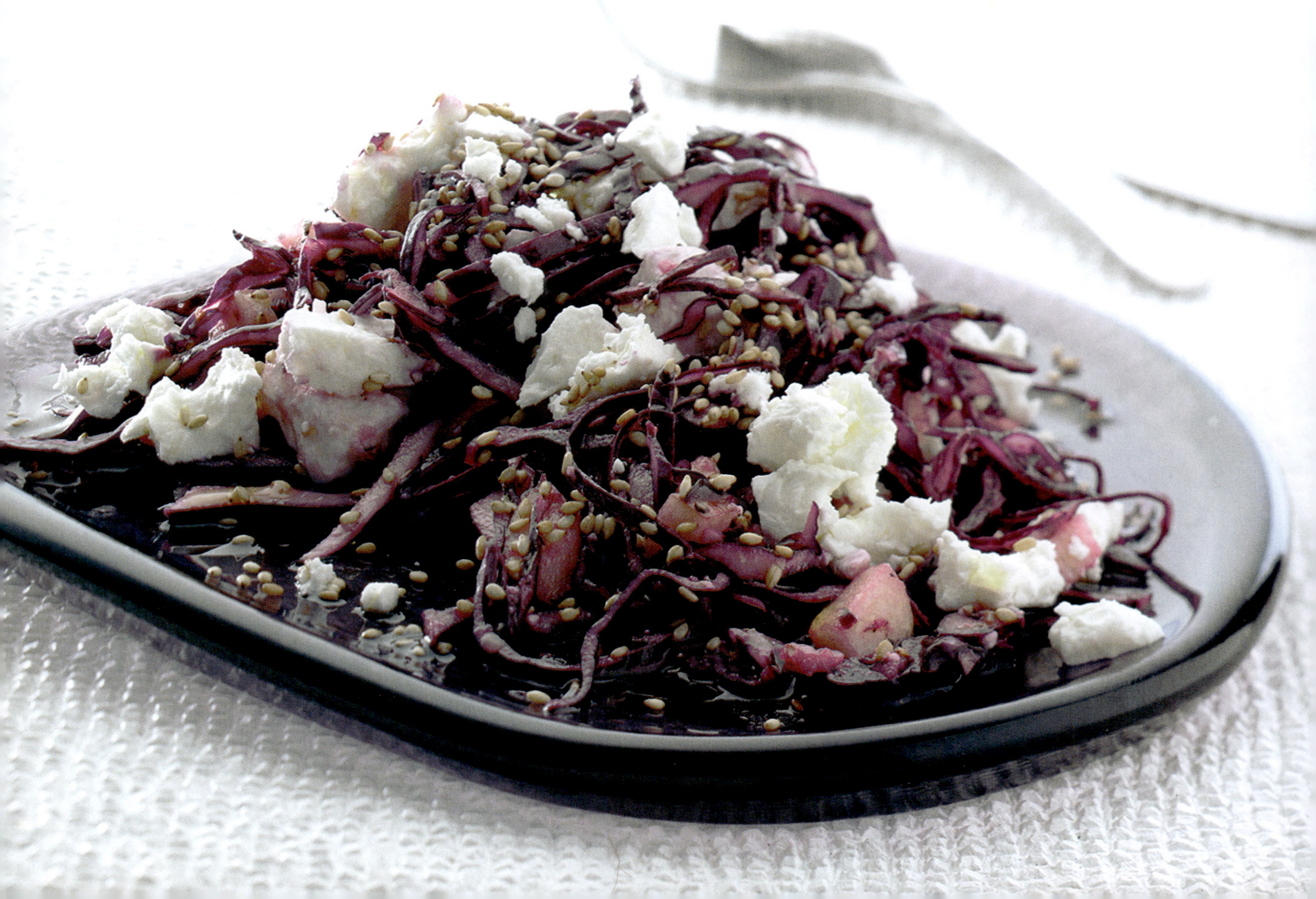

with the olive oil and spices. Do not allow the mixture to brown—if necessary, add a little water. You can add chili powder to taste if you would like the dahl to be hot as well as spicy. Add the lentils, water, and tomatoes. Leave to simmer on a low heat for about 1 hour, stirring regularly to make sure the bottom does not stick. If the dahl starts to become too thick, add a little more water. Serve with brown basmati rice and steamed broccoli.
Serves 3

ROASTED VEGETABLE SALAD

This is a colorful, warming salad that my friend Catherine makes when I visit her in the south of France. The natural sweetness of the potato satisfies any cravings for something stodgy, and you can add other ingredients such as cubed feta cheese, whole-kernel corn, or different vegetables to turn this into a meal in itself.

1 medium-sized sweet potato (preferably the variety with orange flesh)
1 red pepper
1 medium-sized beet (pre-cooked, or peel and roast a fresh one yourself)
2 handfuls of lettuce/rocket/mixed salad leaves
olive oil
balsamic vinegar
salt and pepper

Wash all the vegetables and peel off any bits you don't like the look of from the sweet potato. I tend to leave most of the skin on. Slice the potato into pieces of roughly the same thickness and about 1 inch in diameter. Chop the pepper to the same size. Pour a little olive oil over the sweet-potato and pepper pieces and roast in the oven on a medium/high setting for 30–40 minutes, or until tender and a little crispy round the edges. Chop up the pre-cooked beet into cubes and add to the roasted vegetables. Season and add balsamic vinegar to taste. Serve warm on the salad leaves.
Serves 2

MONGETTES CHARENTAISES

My friend Isabelle first made this for me. Traditionally the dish is served with *gigot d'agneau* (roast lamb). However, I rather like it on its own on a winter's night. The word *mongettes* is the local Charente term for white haricot beans. Traditionally, this should be made from scratch using dried beans that have been soaked and cooked through, but this version is much quicker.

extra-virgin olive oil
2 14-oz (400-g) cans white beans, or fava beans
1 large onion, chopped
2 large tomatoes, chopped
½ empty bean can water
2 cloves garlic, finely chopped
large sprig fresh thyme
2 bay leaves
large pinch sea salt
freshly ground black pepper

Heat the olive oil in a large, heavy saucepan and toss in the beans with the onions and tomatoes, stirring for a few minutes until the onions are soft, but not brown. Add the water, garlic, thyme, bay leaves, salt, and pepper and allow to simmer for about 20 minutes. These beans taste great the next day.
Serves 2, or 4 as a side dish

DUCK-LIVER AND ARTICHOKE SALAD

This dish can be served as a starter at dinner parties, but it also makes a great light supper. I usually use tinned artichoke hearts. Use organic chicken livers if you are unable to find duck livers.

2 large handfuls bitter salad leaves (such as rocket, watercress, endive)
Creamy Vinaigrette (see page 114)
4 artichoke hearts
7 oz (200 g) duck livers
knob of butter
pinch of dried thyme

Tear the salad leaves, toss in the dressing and arrange on the plates. Slice the artichokes and put them on top of the salad. Slice the livers. Heat the butter with the thyme in a non-stick skillet and sauté the livers for a minute or two, until they are firm but not hard. Take them out of the pan with a pancake turner and lay them over the salad. Drizzle with a little more vinaigrette and serve immediately.
Serves 2

JAPANESE-STYLE TUNA SALAD *(below)*

This dish will leave you feeling remarkably satisfied, yet lightly fed, as is the case with most Japanese food. The possible permutations are endless—you can change the marinade to create an entirely different meal. You could also use different types of fish or seafood, such as baby octopus or squid.

¾ lb (350 g) fresh tuna steak
large bunch rocket
½ large cucumber, sliced in long strips
4 scallions, finely sliced
8 cherry tomatoes, halved
1 tablespoon sesame seeds, toasted

For the marinade:
2 tablespoons tamari or soy sauce
1 tablespoon sake/sherry
½ teaspoon wasabi paste

For the dressing:
1 tablespoon lime juice
2 tablespoons tamari or soy sauce
2 teaspoons sesame oil

Mix the tamari, sake, and wasabi in a bowl to make the marinade. Cut up the tuna steak into bite-sized chunks and mix with the marinade. Combine the ingredients for the dressing in a small bowl. Pile the rocket, cucumber strips, sliced scallion, and halved tomatoes on two plates. Heat a griddle pan (or non-stick skillet) and toss the tuna pieces for a few seconds on each side to sear them. Lay them on top of the salad and drizzle with the dressing. Top with the toasted sesame seeds.

Serves 2

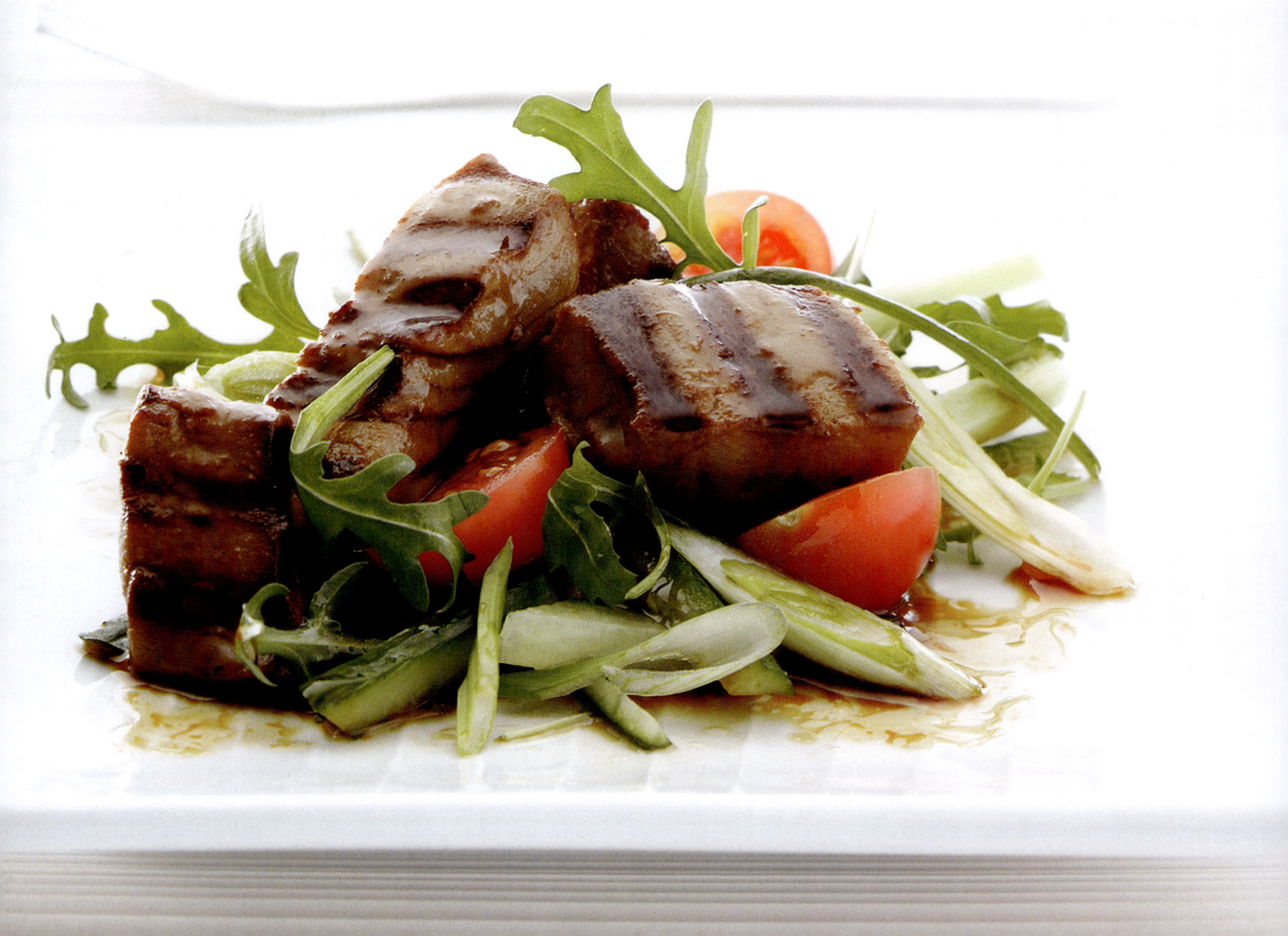

PUY LENTIL SALAD *(below)*

French Puy lentils make a delicious salad—this version looks great, thanks to the contrasting colors. My favorite herb to use in this dish is basil, which evokes the Mediterranean, but you can, if you prefer, use parsley or even fresh coriander. The cold-pressed sunflower oil adds a nutty touch to the lentil mixture. If you can't get hold of cold-pressed sunflower oil, double the amount of olive oil instead—do NOT use common supermarket sunflower oil.

1 cup Puy lentils
3 tomatoes
3 scallions
6 basil leaves
1 tablespoon olive oil
1 tablespoon cold-pressed sunflower oil
2 teaspoons balsamic vinegar
freshly ground black pepper
pinch of salt

Wash the lentils thoroughly and place them in a large pan of cold water. Bring to the boil and simmer until the lentils are cooked. This should take about 30 minutes—taste to check that they are not hard. Drain and leave to cool. While the lentils are cooking, you can pop the tomatoes into the pan for a minute to loosen the skins. Take them out, peel them, and chop them roughly. Then trim and finely slice the scallions and roughly tear the basil leaves. Toss the lentils well with all the other ingredients. I prefer this salad served slightly warm, but it is just as good cold.
Serves 2

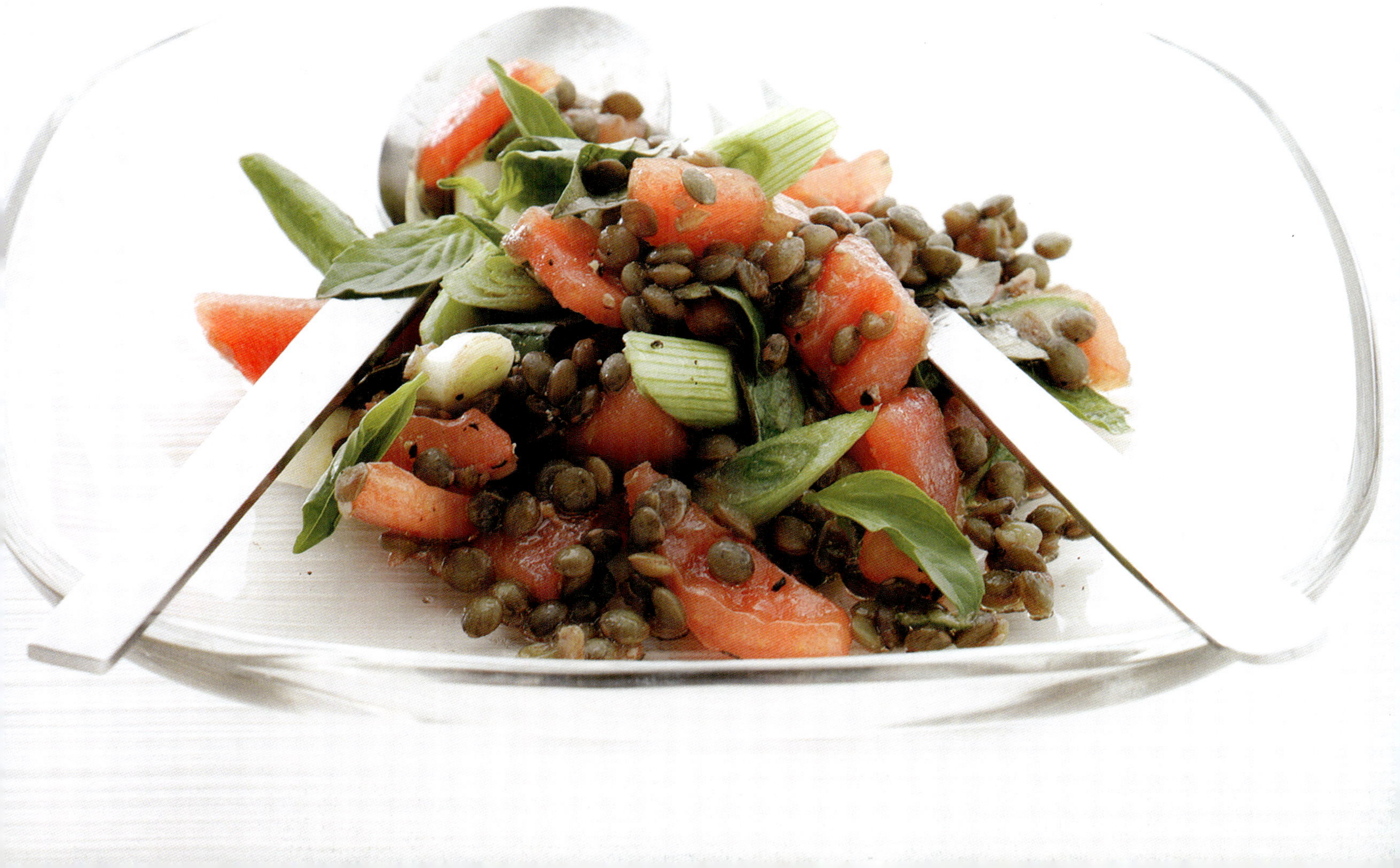

soups

There's nothing like a warming soup in the winter. In fact, all year round soups can make a very satisfying meal. The Thai-Style Noodle Soup on page 96 is definitely a full meal in itself. Other than the Warming Lamb Soup on page 97, all the recipes featured are suitable for vegetarians. I usually make extra soup so that I can freeze some.

Freezing

Make soup with any vegetable, stock and onion. Thicken by cooking it with a potato or a handful of oats. Then puree in a blender, allow to cool, and freeze in sealable containers.

CARROT SOUP *(main image, opposite)*

There are many possible variations on the theme of carrot soup—this is one I made up with flavors from my spice drawer. You can vary it using different spices, such as plain curry powder, or by adding small pieces of lean ham.

1 lb (500 g) carrots
2 sticks celery
1 onion
1 clove garlic
1 teaspoon olive oil
½ teaspoon mustard powder
½ teaspoon wild-onion seeds
2 pinches of salt
dash of Tobasco
sprigs of fresh thyme
½ inch (1¼ cm) grated gingerroot
4 cups (1 l) chicken or vegetable stock
freshly ground black pepper
natural yogurt to serve

Peel and chop the carrots, celery, onion, and garlic. Soften the onion and garlic in a large saucepan with the olive oil and the herbs and spices, adding a couple of tablespoons of the stock after a minute or so. After another 4–5 minutes, add the carrots and celery. Stir well. Pour in the rest of the stock, bring to the boil, then turn down to a simmer and cover. Leave to cook for about 40 minutes. Add more water if the soup thickens too much. When the ingredients are cooked, blend the soup. Serve swirled with a teaspoon of natural yogurt.
Serves 3

CHUNKY VEGETABLE SOUP

This is actually a regular winter veggie soup for which I tend to use stock made from a left-over chicken carcass. You can actually use any vegetables and you can make this soup using a vegetable stock made from powder. The oats make the soup lovely and thick. You can also, if you prefer, puree it in a blender.

4 cups (1 l) stock
2 onions
2 carrots
2 sticks celery
1 leek
½ turnip
5–6 collard-green leaves
1 teaspoon olive oil
3–4 sprigs fresh thyme
½ teaspoon dried, mixed herbs
1 tablespoon oats
freshly ground black pepper
pinch of salt

If you're making stock, put the chicken carcass in a large saucepan with 6 cups (1½ l) water, an onion, a few peppercorns, fresh thyme, and a half teaspoon of salt. Leave to simmer for 2 hours and then strain, discarding the bits. Otherwise, you can use ready-made stock or stock cubes. Next, prepare the vegetables: Peel and chop the onion; peel and slice the carrots; trim and slice the celery; trim and slice the leek; peel and dice the turnip; and trim the tough ends from the collard-green leaves. Heat the olive oil in a large saucepan and add the vegetables one by one, onions first. Stir well, adding the herbs. Stir in the oats and pour the stock into the pan, adding freshly ground black pepper and a pinch of salt. Leave to simmer for at least 45 minutes. Either serve as it is—a rough, veggie soup—or put in a blender to make a smooth, pureed soup.
Serves 3

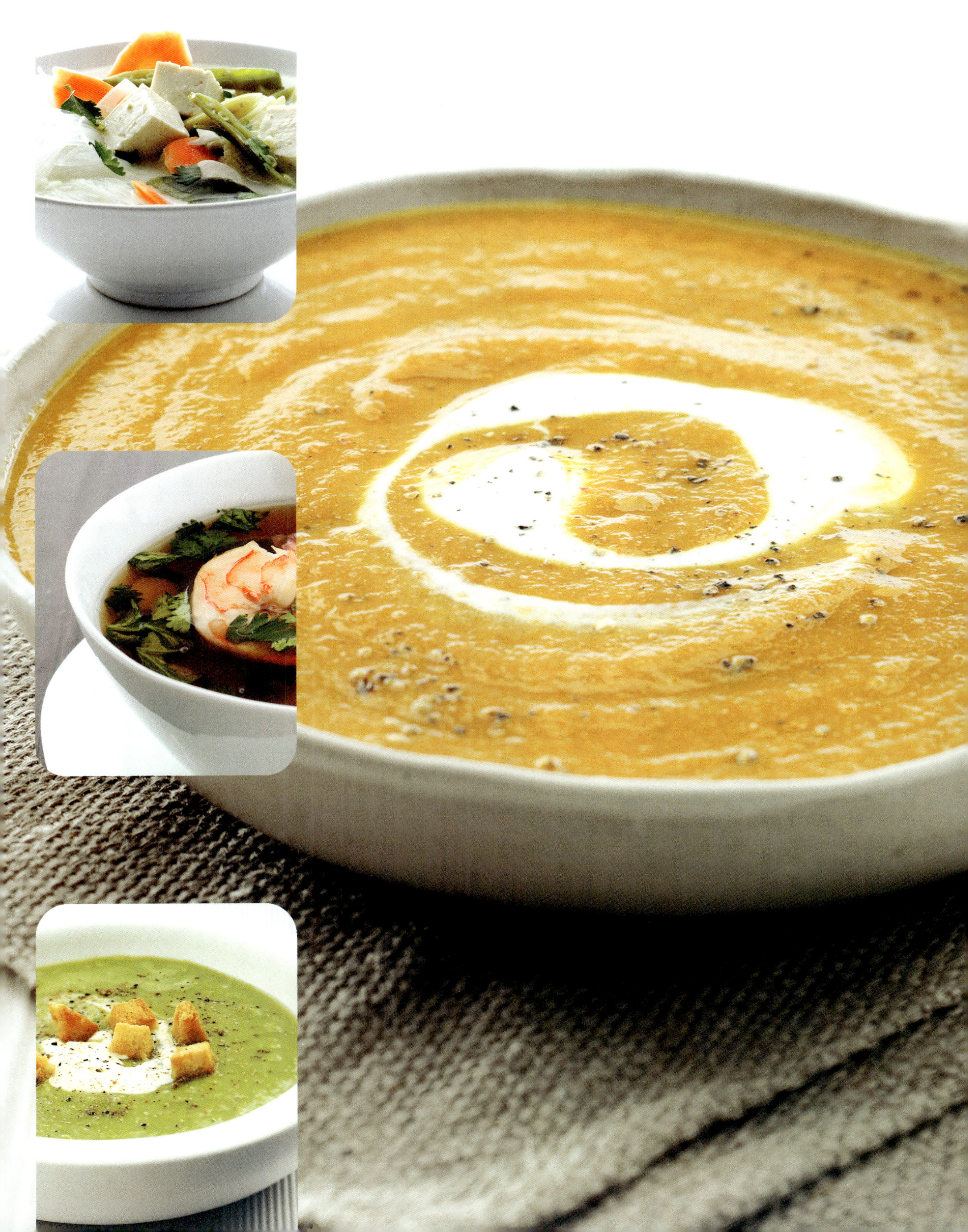

THAI-STYLE NOODLE SOUP *(below)*

There are so many variations on the theme of Asian-style soups that you can experiment with: hotter, vegetarian, with or without noodles. This recipe is for a filling meal in itself—you can substitute the shrimps with slices of fish, chicken breast, beef, or tofu. If you decide to make extra for freezing, don't do the noodles for the frozen batch. Instead, cook them at the last minute when you're serving it.

5 oz (150 g) vermicelli rice noodles
1 stick lemon grass
2 cloves garlic
1 inch (2½ cm) gingerroot
8 sticks baby corn
8 scallions
sprigs fresh coriander
extra-virgin olive oil
2 teaspoons Thai green curry paste
9 oz (250 g) fresh shrimps or tofu, etc.
1 14-fl oz (400-ml) can coconut milk
3–4 kaffir-lime leaves
2 carrots, peeled
12 snow peas

Cook the rice noodles as directed on the packet, rinse well with cold water, and divide between four large bowls.

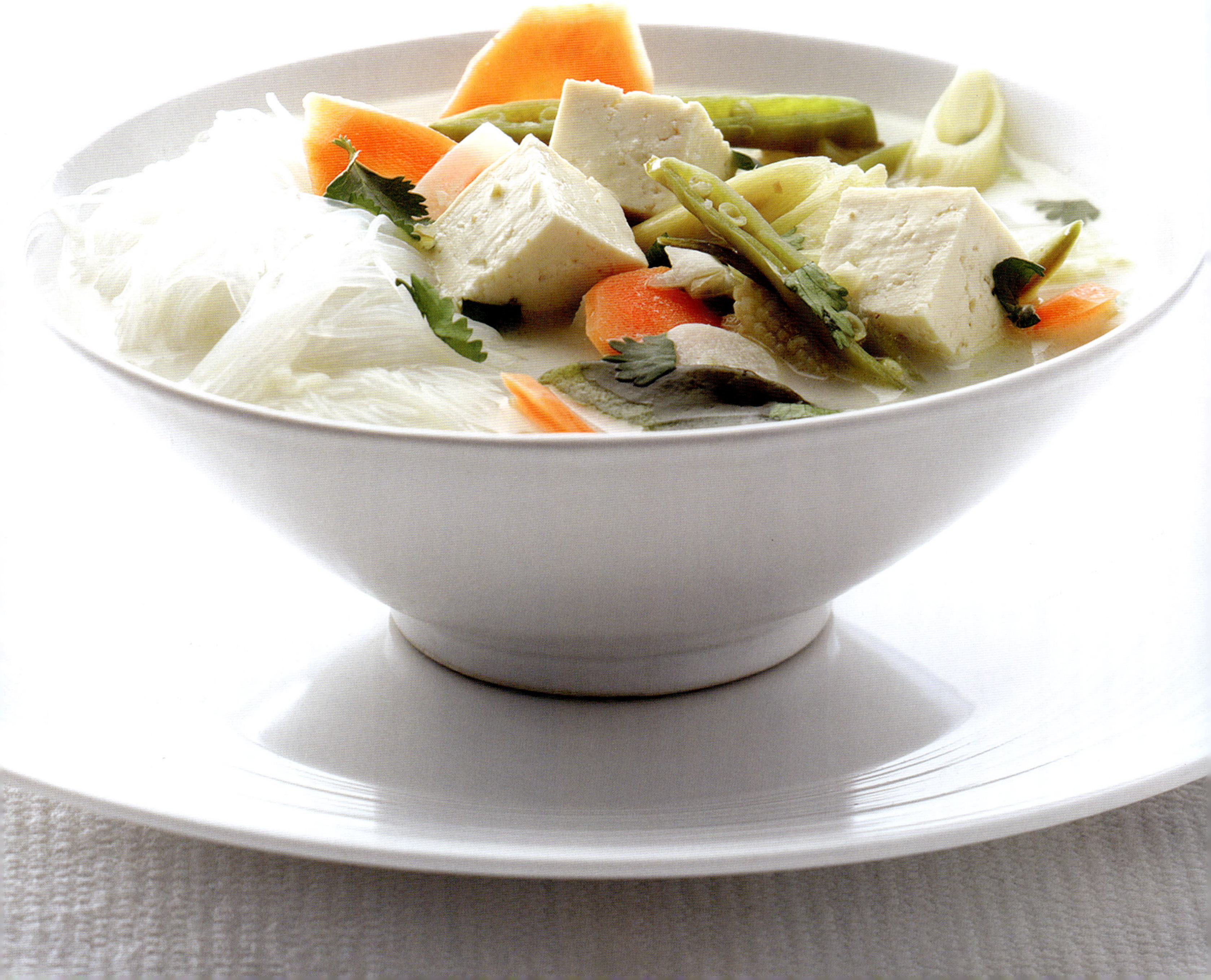

Prepare the vegetables: Slice the lemon grass into about six pieces; chop the garlic finely; slice the gingerroot, baby corn, scallions, and carrots; and chop the coriander.

In a large pan, heat the olive oil and stir in the curry paste, chopped garlic, sliced lemon grass, and sliced gingerroot. Add a tablespoon of water. Toss in the shrimps and stir for a few minutes until they are pink and cooked through. Fish them out with a slotted spoon and lay them on the noodles.

Add the rest of the vegetables, including the snow peas, to the pan, stirring them in the spices for a couple of minutes. Pour in the coconut milk and add the kaffir-lime leaves. Add a couple of canfuls of water, bring to the boil, and leave to simmer for 12–15 minutes, or until the vegetables are cooked. At the last minute, stir in half the chopped coriander. Ladle the soup evenly over the noodles and cooked shrimps and garnish with the rest of the fresh coriander.

Serves 4

LEEK AND POTATO SOUP

My Aunt Claire first gave me this recipe when I was a student—it is economical, filling and delicious, not to mention easy to make. It can be eaten hot or cold.

3 medium-sized leeks
1 large potato
½ medium-sized onion, peeled
1 clove garlic
2½ cups (600 ml) vegetable stock
1 *bouquet garni*
1 teaspoon olive oil
black pepper
2 teaspoons tamari or soy sauce
4 teaspoons natural yogurt or quark

First wash the leeks thoroughly. I find the best way to get all the soil out of them without wastage is to trim off and discard both ends. Then slice the whole leek down the middle lengthways, slice crossways, and rinse in a sieve. Roughly chop the potato and peeled onion. Crush the garlic. Make up the stock using a vegetable stock powder. Soften the onions and garlic in the olive oil, adding the washed leeks, potatoes, and 3 tablespoons of the stock. Pour in the rest of the stock, add the *bouquet garni*, and season with freshly ground black pepper and the tamari or soy sauce. Cover and leave to simmer until the potatoes are soft (at least 25 minutes). Pour into a blender and mix until smooth. Before serving, swirl a teaspoon of natural yogurt in each bowl.

Serves 3

FISH SOUP PROVENÇALE

My friend Catherine who lives in the south of France gave me this version of a local dish. The best flavor comes from making your own stock using fish heads, but ready-made or a stock cube will do.

1 medium-sized onion
2 cloves garlic
1 medium-sized zucchini
15–20 scarlet runner beans
1 stick celery
1 teaspoon olive oil
2½ cups (600 ml) fish stock
1 tablespoon tomato paste
1 teaspoon thyme (or two fresh stalks)
1 teaspoon oregano
freshly ground black pepper
pinch salt
4 oz (100 g) white fish, such as haddock, monkfish
2 oz (50 g) mussels (frozen are probably easiest)
2 oz (50 g) shrimps
1 tablespoon chopped parsley

Finely chop the onion, garlic, zucchini, beans, and celery.

Soften the onion and garlic in the olive oil and 2 tablespoons of the fish stock. Add the tomato paste and stir well. Add the zucchini, beans, celery, thyme, and oregano. Pour in the rest of the stock, season and cover to simmer for 30 minutes. Cube the white fish and add to the soup with the mussels and shrimps. Leave to cook for 5 minutes. Discard any unopened mussel shells. Just before serving, sprinkle with the freshly chopped parsley.

Serves 2–3

WARMING LAMB SOUP

This is one of my favorite cold-weather soups. And because you can use ready-made stock and canned beans (any will do), it really doesn't take long to prepare.

continued

4 cups (1 l) lamb stock
1 large onion
2 cloves garlic
1 stick celery
1 medium-sized carrot
1 14-oz (400-g) can lima beans or other
3–4 sprigs fresh thyme
2 teaspoons oatmeal oats
1 teaspoon olive oil
freshly ground black pepper
pinch of salt

Either buy ready-made lamb stock, or, ideally, simmer lamb bones with a handful of thyme and an onion for 2 hours and skim the fat from the top before making the soup. You can use home-made or bought chicken stock instead if you prefer.

For the soup, peel and chop the onion and garlic. Slice the celery and carrot. Soften the onion in the olive oil and a tablespoon of the stock. Add the celery, carrot, oats, fresh thyme, and lima beans and stir well. Season with plenty of freshly ground black pepper and a pinch of salt. Add the rest of the stock and leave to simmer for half an hour. I prefer the texture of the soup as it is—with all its identifiable lumps—but if you prefer, put the mixture in a blender and whizz it until it is smooth. Serve piping hot.
Serves 4

BEAN AND ZUCCHINI SOUP

This is a variation on a *pistou*, or pesto, soup made in France.

1 medium-sized onion, peeled and sliced
2 cups (250 g) scarlet runner beans, washed and sliced
2 14-oz (420-g) cans haricot beans
2 large zucchini, washed and sliced
3 cloves garlic
bunch of fresh basil
3 medium-sized tomatoes, peeled and chopped
freshly ground black pepper
pinch of sea salt
1 tablespoon freshly grated Parmesan cheese
olive oil
2 pt (1 l) water

In a large pan, soften the onion in half a tablespoon of olive oil. Add the scarlet runner and haricot beans and zucchini and stir for a few minutes. Cover with water. While this is cooking, put the garlic, basil leaves, tomatoes, salt and pepper, and a tablespoon of grated Parmesan in a blender, slowly adding about a tablespoon of olive oil to make a pesto sauce. Hold back a few basil leaves for garnishing. Check the vegetables are well cooked—this should take about 20 minutes. If the soup gets too thick, add a little more water. Just before serving, pour the pesto into the soup and stir well.To serve, grate some more Parmesan on each bowlful and top with a basil leaf.
Serves 3–4

HOT AND SOUR SOUP

(opposite)

This is a version of the sharp Thai soup called Tom Yum Goong. You can use any other fish, or even chicken or tofu instead of the shrimps. Although the list of ingredients may seem long, this soup really takes no time at all to prepare. It's best to use home-made fish stock, prepared by boiling fish bones with lemon grass, chili, kaffir-lime leaves, and galangal (in which case don't use the lime leaves or galangal in the soup), but if you don't have the time or inclination, just use stock cubes. To make a more filling soup, you could add rice noodles.

1 lb (500 g) uncooked shrimps
2 small red, fresh chilies
1 stick of lemon grass, sliced
1 inch (2½ cm) gingerroot, grated
3 dried kaffir-lime leaves
3 sliced dried galangal
1 tablespoon fresh lime juice
2 teaspoons brown sugar
4 scallions, sliced
1 14-oz (400-g) can straw mushrooms, drained
1 tablespoon fish sauce
1 tablespoon tamari or soy sauce
6 cups (1½ l) fish stock
fresh coriander to garnish

If you have bought whole shrimps, shell them, leaving the tails on. Put the shrimps, chilies, lemon grass, ginger, kaffir-lime leaves, galangal, lime juice, sugar, scallions, mushrooms, fish sauce, and tamari or soy sauce into the stock. Bring it to the boil and then simmer until the shrimps are cooked through. Garnish with fresh coriander.
Serves 4

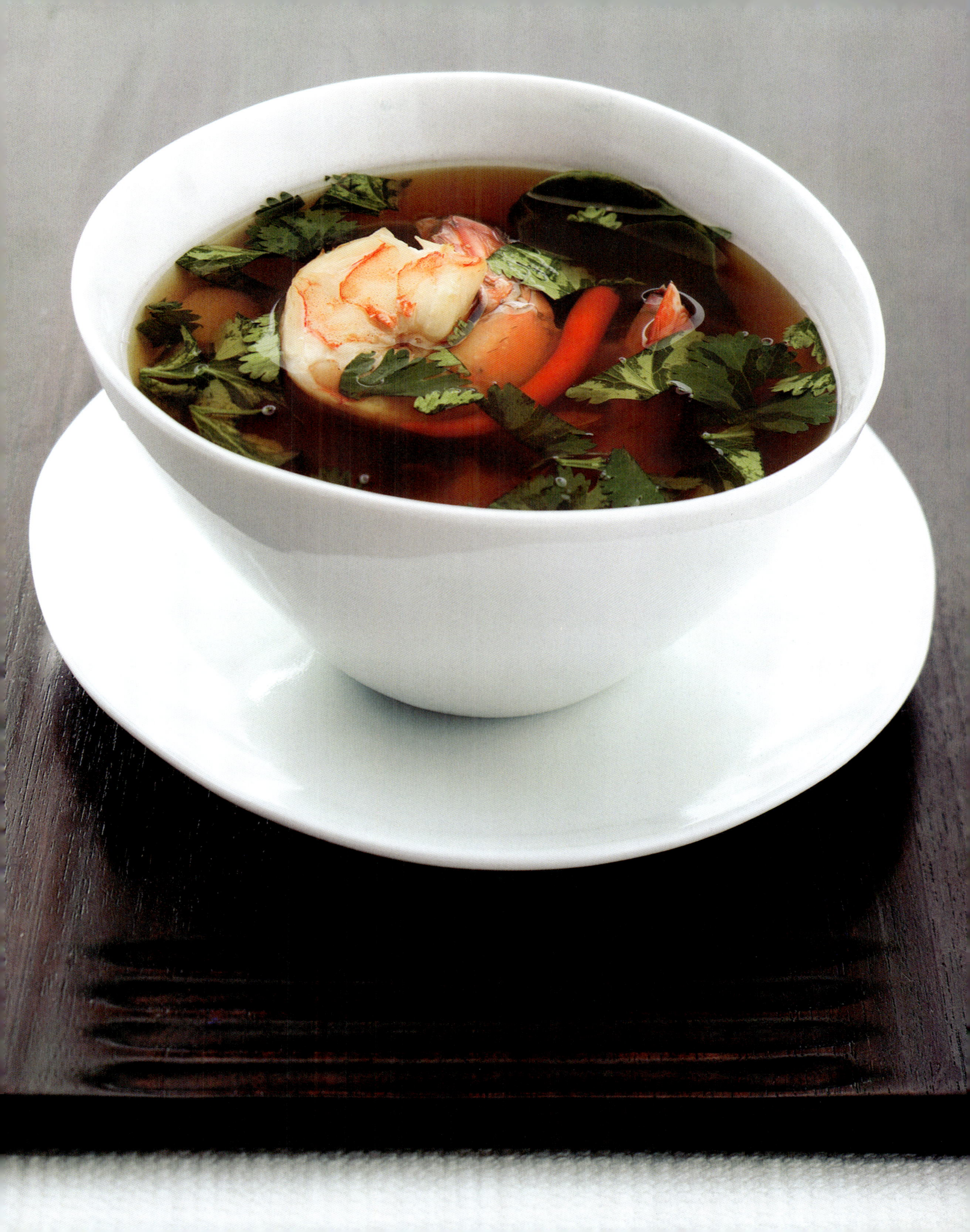

main meals

With flavors from far and wide, these recipes provide the focal dish of a lunchtime or evening meal, even when you are entertaining. Try to use only fresh ingredients, and feel free to play around with permutations that appeal more to your palate.

You can serve these main meals with the suggested accompaniment or browse through the recipes for side dishes and salads on pages 114–117.

STUFFED VEGETABLES

This makes a satisfying supper. It can also serve as a good main course for a vegetarian if you leave out the turkey and add a can of beans (for example, pinto) instead. If you like large zucchini, they contrast well with eggplants.

2 large eggplants or 1 eggplant and 1 large zucchini
1 medium-sized onion
1 stick celery
2 teaspoons olive oil
1 tablespoon water
9 oz (250 g) turkey mince
⅓ cup (50 g) brown and wild rice (cooked)
1 clove garlic
1 large tomato, peeled
2 oz (50 g) goat's cheddar (or feta)

Preheat the oven to 350°F/gas mark 4. Slice the eggplants and/or zucchini lengthways, carefully cutting through the stalks so that half of the stalk remains on each piece (this makes the halved vegetables look more attractive). Scoop out the flesh, leaving about ½ inch (1 cm) of flesh inside the skin. Set the skins aside. Finely chop the eggplant (and zucchini) flesh, the peeled onion, and celery.

Soften the vegetables in the olive oil and water over a low heat—after a few minutes, add the turkey and stir well. Add the cooked rice. Crush the garlic and chop the tomato and stir into the pan with the other ingredients. Grate the goat's cheddar (or crumble the feta) and fold into the mixture, holding back a couple of spoonfuls. Fill the empty eggplant skins with the mixture, top with the remaining grated or crumbled cheese, and bake in the oven for 1 hour.
Serves 4

FRITTATA *(main image, opposite)*

This is a versatile, delicious meal and can be made to be eaten later or the next day. A slice also makes a good centerpiece for a packed lunch. You can replace one of the zucchini with a red pepper if you prefer, although I'm not a fan of egg and pepper together. Eggs are a great source of protein and a range of other nutrients, especially for vegetarians.

5 oz (150 g) new potatoes
1 red onion
2 zucchini
1 tablespoon olive oil
sprig of fresh thyme
salt
freshly ground black pepper
6 medium-sized eggs

Wash the potatoes, quarter them, and boil them until tender. Slice the onion and washed zucchini finely. Heat the oil in a large pan and soften the onion for 2–3 minutes without allowing it to brown. Add the zucchini, a pinch of salt, the thyme (leaves scraped from the twigs), and freshly ground black pepper. Cook for another 3 minutes.

Stir in the cooked potatoes and remove the pan from the heat. Beat the eggs. Although you can beat all six eggs together, the fluffiest frittata is made by beating four of the eggs, whole and whisking the whites of the other two, and then folding the whites into the other eggs. Preheat the grill. Pour the egg mixture into the pan with the vegetables. Cook on a very low heat for about 8 minutes, until the eggs are nearly set. Place the pan under the grill and cook until the eggs are completely set. Using a pancake turner, cut the frittata into generous wedges. You can serve it as it is, warm, or later, cold. Serve with Proper Green Salad (see page 114) or Wild Tomato Salad (see page 117).
serves 4

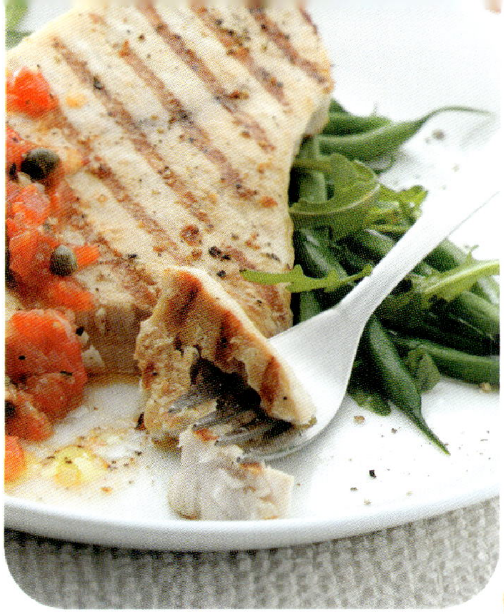
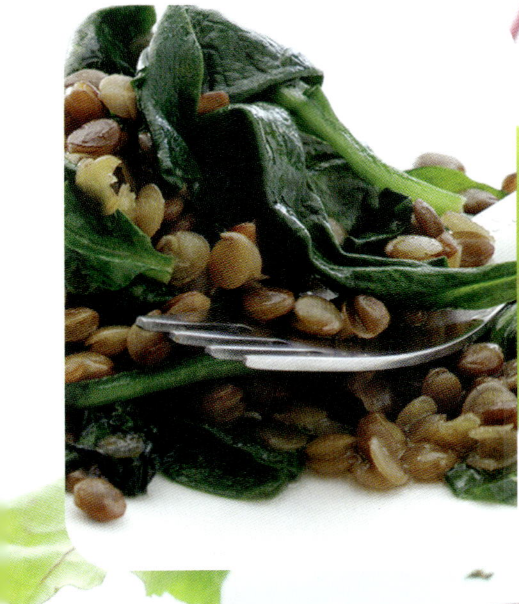
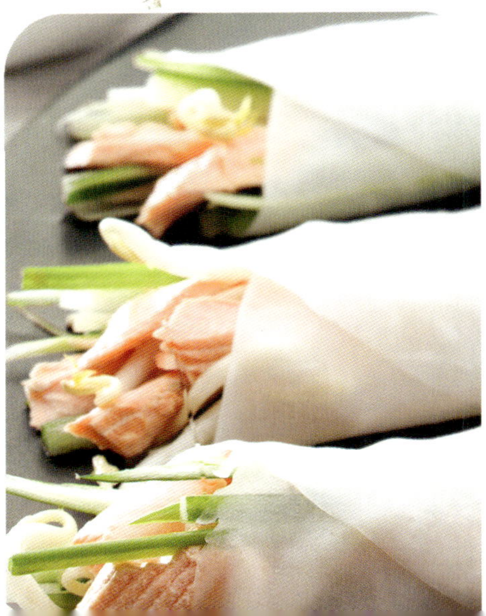
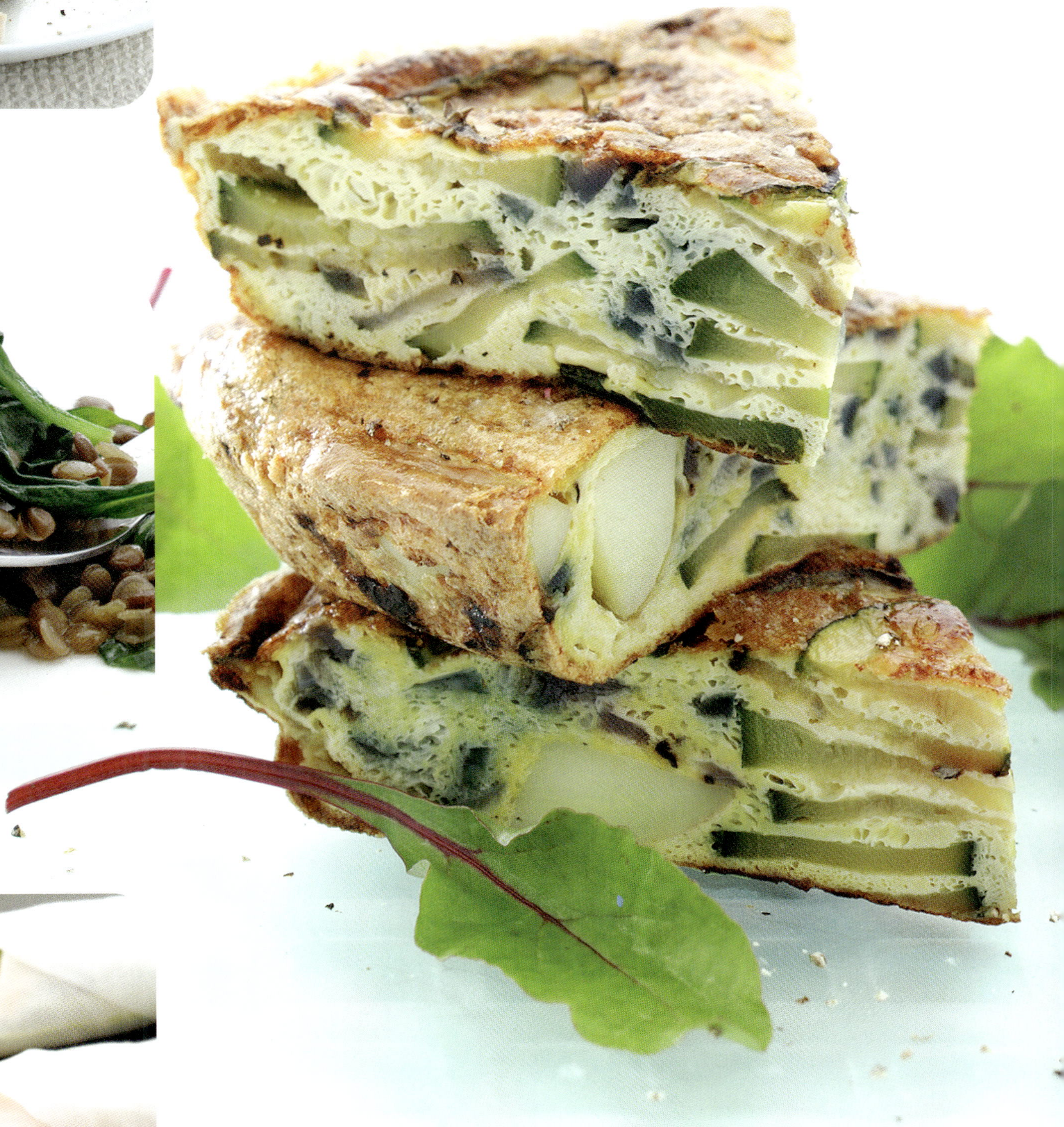

FISH STEW PROVENÇALE

The recipe for Fish Soup on page 97 can be easily converted to a thicker fish *ragoût*, or stew, and served as a main dish. To do so:

Halve the amount of fish stock to 1½ cups (300 ml), or ¾ cups (200 ml) and ½ cup (100 ml) of white wine. Add 1 14-oz (400-g) can of chopped, canned tomatoes when you put in the vegetables, and add a handful of squid rings along with the fish. Serve with brown rice.

Serves 4

KEBABS

Skewered, broiled fish makes a healthy, easy meal that takes no time to prepare. You can vary the kebabs by using different fish or meats, a variety of vegetables and—my sneaky way of varying very similar dishes—the marinade. If you like, swap the fish for chicken and lamb pieces. Serve with brown basmati rice and a green salad and you could be in the Middle East.

7 oz (200 g) monkfish
7 oz (200 g) salmon
4 scallops
4 large shrimps
2 zucchini
1 red pepper
1 yellow pepper
4 bamboo skewers

For the marinade:
juice of 3 limes
freshly ground black pepper
3 tablespoons olive oil
½ teaspoon ground turmeric
½ teaspoon ground coriander
1 teaspoon Tobasco sauce
pinch of salt
sprigs of fresh parsley to garnish

Cut the monkfish and salmon into four equal-sized cubes. In a large dish, mix all the marinade ingredients and add the fish, scallops, and shrimps, coating them well. Leave them to stand, ideally for an hour. Meanwhile, if you are using wooden skewers soak them in cold water to prevent them from burning.

Slice the zucchini crossways. Deseed the peppers and cut them into 1-inch (2½-cm) square pieces. Prepare the skewers, separating each piece of fish with vegetables. Broil the kebabs until the fish is cooked—this should take no longer than 12 minutes. Half way through cooking, turn and baste with the remainder of the marinade.

Serve on a bed of rice garnished with parsley and accompanied by a large, green salad. The rice is tastier if it is cooked in fish stock instead of plain water.

Serves 4

For a more Western Mediterranean-style marinade:
3 tablespoons olive oil
juice of 2 lemons
1 teaspoon fresh thyme leaves
8 large basil leaves, roughly torn
freshly ground black pepper
pinch of salt
a few capers to garnish

For an Indian-style marinade:
⅔ cup (150 g) natural yogurt
1 teaspoon ground coriander
½ teaspoon ground cumin
½ teaspoon turmeric powder
½ onion, grated
pinch of salt
freshly ground black pepper

For a Far Eastern-style marinade:
1 tablespoon sesame oil
juice of 3 limes
2 fresh chilies, finely chopped
2 cloves garlic, crushed
1 tablespoon fish sauce
1 inch (2½ cm) fresh gingerroot, grated

BROILED SWORDFISH IN CAPER SALSA *(opposite)*

My sister, Arielle, can rustle this dish up in no time at all, even after a busy day at work. For both Arielle and myself, the combination of fresh swordfish and capers evokes wonderful summer-time open-air lunches in Malta; capers grow almost like weeds there, hanging from ancient bastions and creeping through the rocks. In this delicious dish you will find that the capers provide a distinctive flavor.

2 large tomatoes
3 small shallots
1 teaspoon olive oil
1 tablespoon capers
juice of 1 lime
4 swordfish steaks
olive oil to baste

Peel, deseed, and roughly chop the tomatoes. You can drop them in boiling water for a minute to make them easier to peel. Chop the shallots very finely.

Heat the shallots in the olive oil in a small saucepan. When the shallots are soft (do not allow them to brown) add the chopped tomatoes, capers, and lime juice and stir the mixture for just a couple of minutes as it warms through. Remove from the heat while you cook the fish. Brush the fish steaks with olive oil and place under a grill. Cooking should take 12–15 minutes—turn them over half way through. Alternatively, you can cook the fish in a griddle pan. Serve topped with the warm salsa.

Serves 4

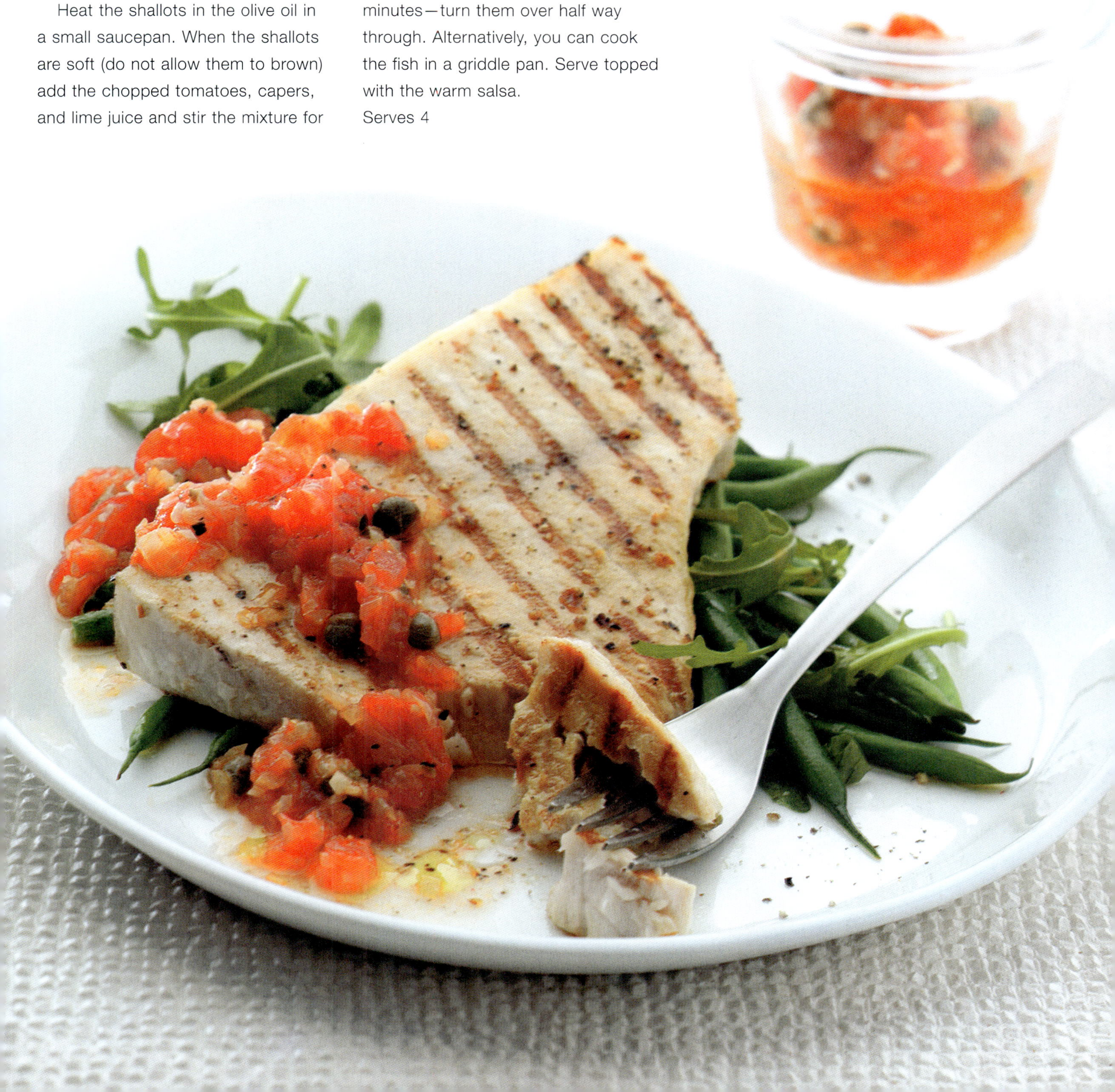

BROILED RAINBOW TROUT *(below)*

My sister Arielle gave me this simple but delicious recipe. What I love about this dish is the fact that you can pick up the ingredients from the supermarket after work, and toss them together in a few minutes.

4 fillets of rainbow trout, washed and dried
6 fl oz (200 ml) low-fat crème fraîche
4 oz (100 g) ready-cooked shrimps
1 bunch chives

Place the fish fillets under a preheated grill for 2–3 minutes on each side. In a saucepan, heat the crème fraîche along with the chives and shrimps. Put each of the pieces of rainbow trout on a plate and pour the sauce over them.

Serve with a Proper Green Salad (see page 114), boiled new potatoes, and steamed broccoli.
Serves 4

TROUT WITH SUNFLOWER SEEDS

This is a wonderful variation on a classic dinner-party dish—trout with almonds. You can use any fish you like instead of trout, but do make sure that it is fresh.

4 trout, gutted, head on
2 lemons
3 tablespoons sunflower seeds
1 tablespoon olive oil

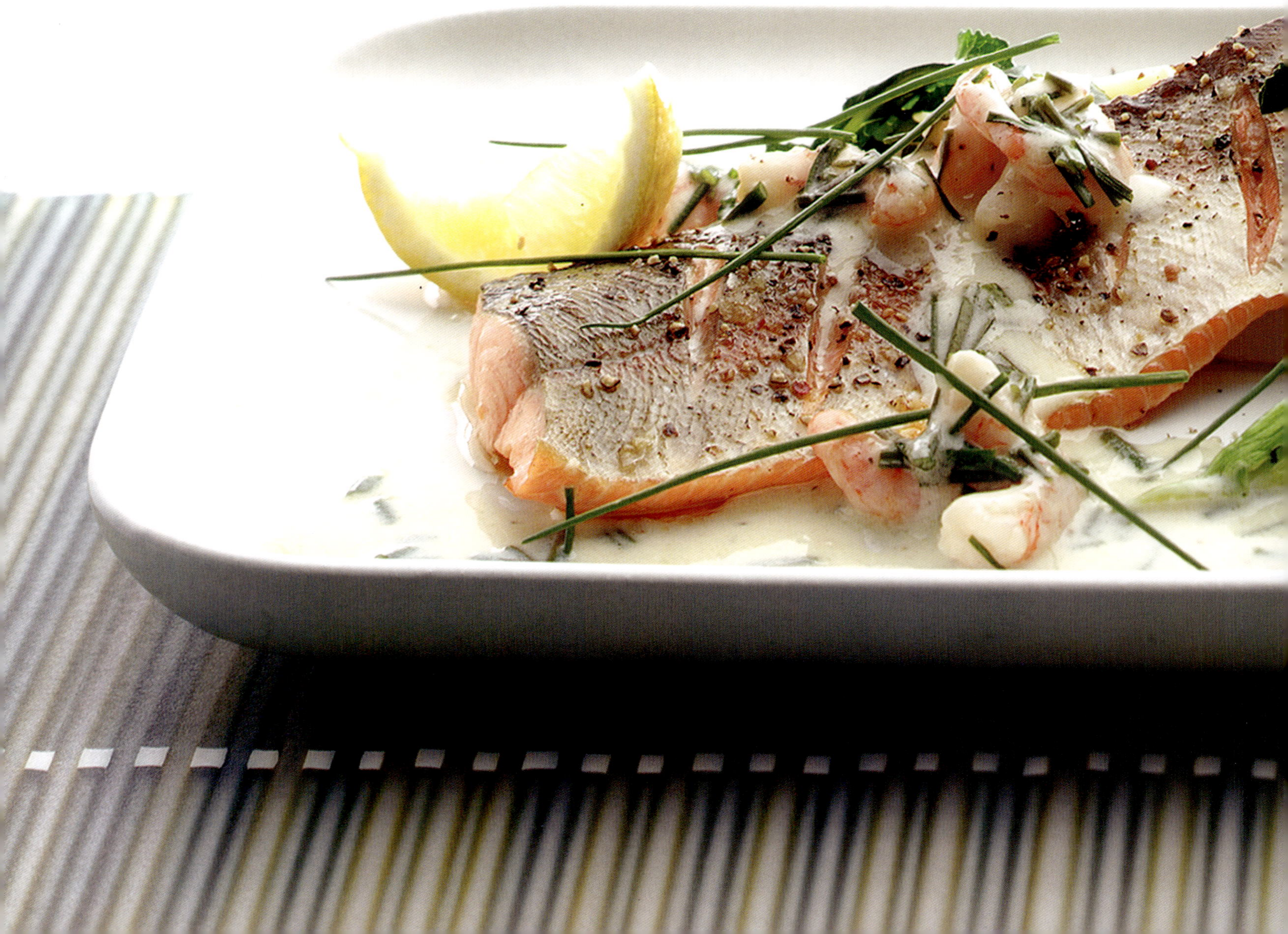

Lay the gutted and rinsed fish in an oven-proof baking dish. Cut the lemons in half and squeeze the juice over the fish. Drizzle the olive oil over the trout. Place in the oven and bake for 20 minutes at 400°F/gas mark 6, turning them over once half way through cooking.

Toss the sunflower seeds in a dry skillet until they are lightly toasted. Just before serving the fish, sprinkle the seeds over the top of each trout. Serves 4

BROILED MACKEREL ON A BED OF STINGING NETTLES

My friend James Verner gave me this exotic recipe. Be brave—put on a pair of gloves and pick those nettles (just the tender leaves at the tips).

5 red chilis
1 clove garlic
a handful of a mixture of fresh sage, thyme, and parsley
3 tablespoons olive oil
4 mackerel, gutted, head on
25 stinging-nettle tips
balsamic vinegar
4 slices of lemon

Mash 1 chili, the garlic, and the herbs with the olive oil in a pestle and mortar. Place this mixture inside the fish and secure with a cocktail stick. Steam the nettles until they lose their sting—this takes about 5 minutes. While steaming the nettles, put the mackerel under a hot grill for about 3–4 minutes per side. Really fresh fish can be left slightly underdone. Toss the nettles in olive oil and lay them on the plates.

Put a fish on top of each bed of nettles and splash on some balsamic vinegar. Garnish with a twist of lemon and a whole chili.

If you cannot steam the nettles, merely rinse them in water and put them in a saucepan to cook like spinach. Drink the remaining liquid, which cleanses the digestive system. Serves 4

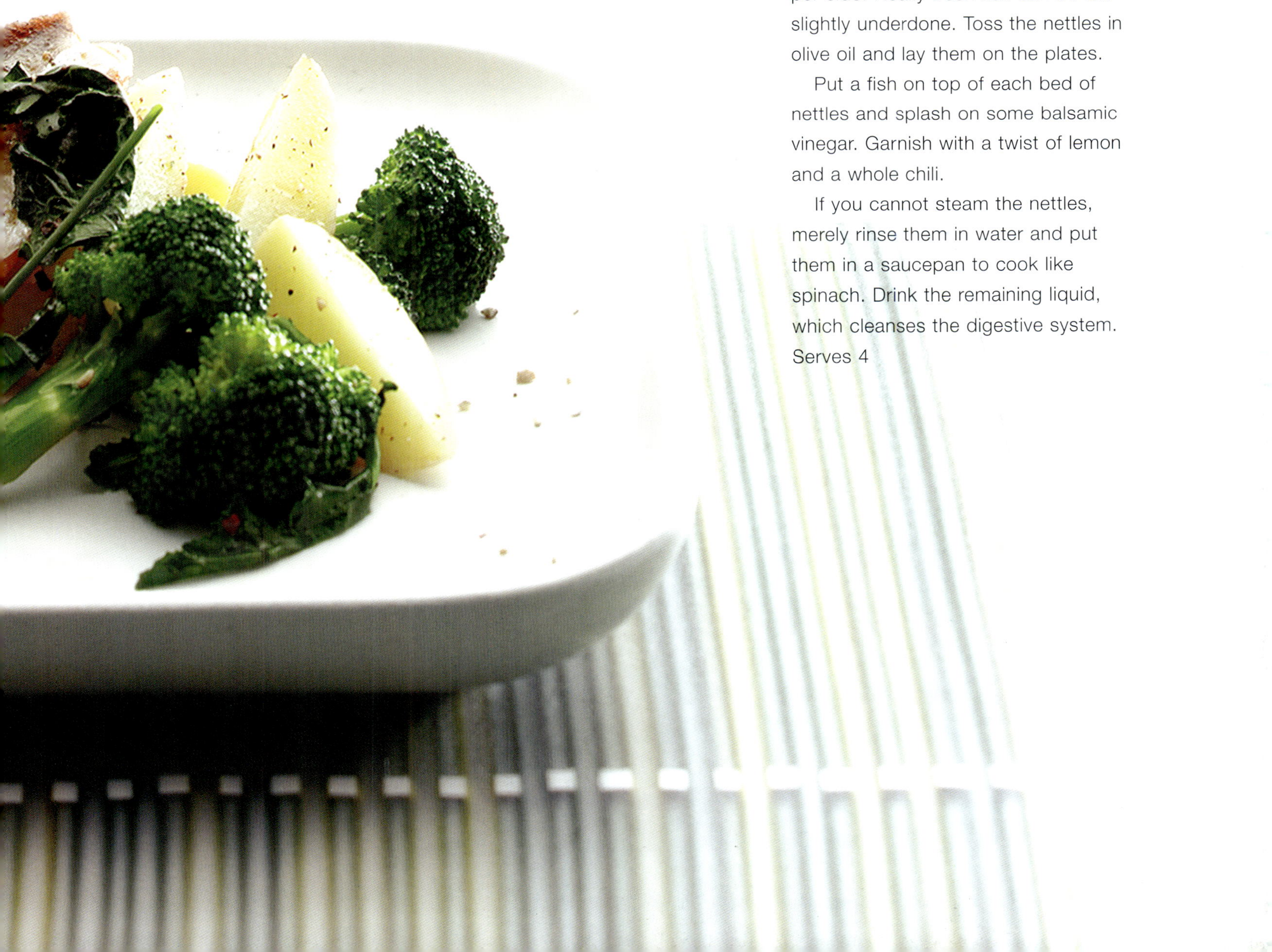

SALMON ROLLS *(opposite)*

I suppose these rolls were initially inspired by a cross between Vietnamese spring rolls and Chinese crispy-duck pancakes! As well as tasting fantastic, the rolls are a fun way to share food around a table with friends. If you cannot find or cannot be bothered with the actual pancakes themselves, you can roll the salmon filling in large lettuce leaves instead.

4 salmon fillet steaks
1 cucumber
4–6 scallions
large handful of bean sprouts
8–10 tablespoons tamari or soy sauce
1 inch (2½ cm) gingerroot, grated
3 tablespoons toasted sesame oil
at least 16 rice pancakes

Steam or poach the salmon. When it is cooked, roughly break it up with a fork and leave it to cool in a serving bowl. Slice the cucumber and scallions into long, thin strips and arrange them with the bean sprouts on a serving plate.

Mix the tamari or soy sauce, grated ginger, and sesame oil in two small serving bowls. Prepare the pancakes as directed on the packet. Put the serving bowls on the table and get people to roll some salmon and vegetables in a pancake (or large lettuce leaf) and, using their hands, dip it into the sauce before eating it.

Served with stir-fried vegetables and plain rice, these rolls make a great focus for a dinner party.
Serves 4

SESAME STIR-FRY

This chicken-and-vegetable stir-fry is fabulous served on top of rice noodles and sprinkled with sesame seeds.

2 chicken breasts, lean and skinless, or about 6 oz (180 g) shrimps or beef
1 tablespoon soy sauce
½ inch (1¼ cm) gingerroot, finely sliced
1 clove garlic, finely sliced
1 tablespoon olive oil
1 teaspoon Chinese Five Spice
a handful of sugar snap peas or snow peas
1 onion, chopped
1 red pepper, cut into strips
1 carrot, cut into thin strips
1 tablespoon fresh coriander, finely chopped
2 tablespoons sesame seeds

Slice the chicken (or shrimps or beef) into thin strips and mix well in a bowl along with the soy sauce, sliced ginger, and sliced garlic.

Heat a wok or frying pan and add half a tablespoon of the olive oil. Quickly stir in the marinated chicken, with the sauce, garlic, and ginger, tossing continuously until the chicken is cooked through. Remove the chicken with a slotted spoon (leaving any liquid in the pan), and put aside.

Add the other dessertspoon of olive oil to the pan to heat. Put the Chinese Five Spice and all the prepared vegetables into the pan. Toss quickly and add 2 tablespoons of water to "steam fry." Stir well on a high heat for about 2 minutes. Then put the chicken back into the pan and reheat until you are sure it is hot all the way, without letting the vegetables become soft.
Serves 4

THAI-STYLE ICEFISH

You can use any white fish for this dish, but my favorite is the delicious, rich Antartic icefish (or sea bass).

1 inch (2½ cm) fresh gingerroot
2 cloves garlic
1 lime
2 teaspoons tamari or soy sauce
Tobasco sauce
4 white fish steaks

Grate the ginger, garlic, and the zest of the lime into an ovenproof baking dish. Squeeze in the juice of the lime, along with the tamari or soy sauce and 3–4 dashes of Tobasco sauce and stir well.

Wash the fish steaks and dry them on paper towels. Place them in the baking dish and coat with the marinade. Ideally, marinate the fish for a couple of hours, but this is not essential. Heat the oven to 400°F/gas mark 6. Add 4 tablespoons of water to the fish and mix it well with the marinade before putting the dish into the oven. Bake for 20 minutes or until the fish is cooked through. (The icefish usually takes longer to cook than most white fish as it is very dense.)

Serve with steamed or stir-fried vegetables and brown rice or Roasted Sweet Vegetables (see page 117).
Serves 4

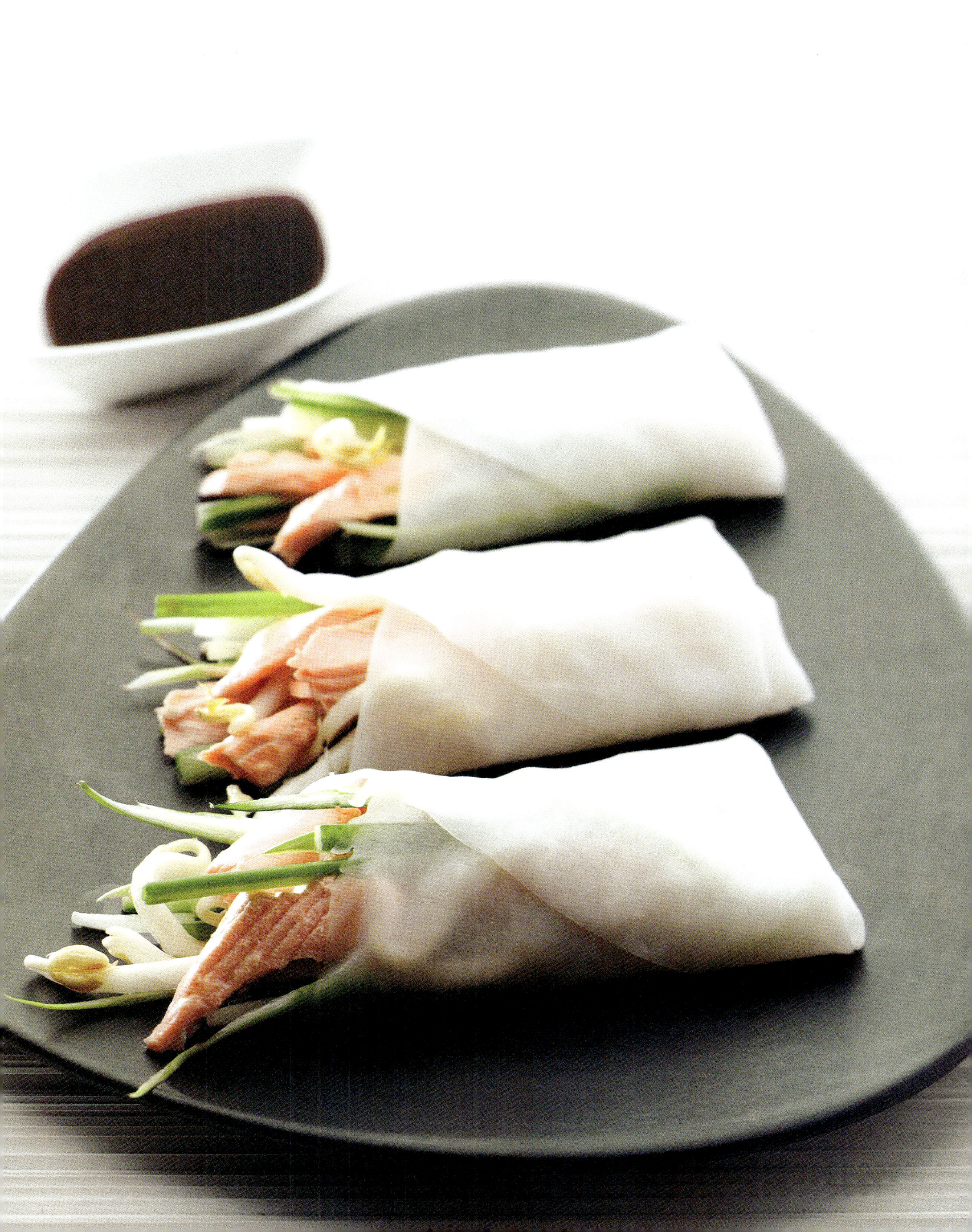

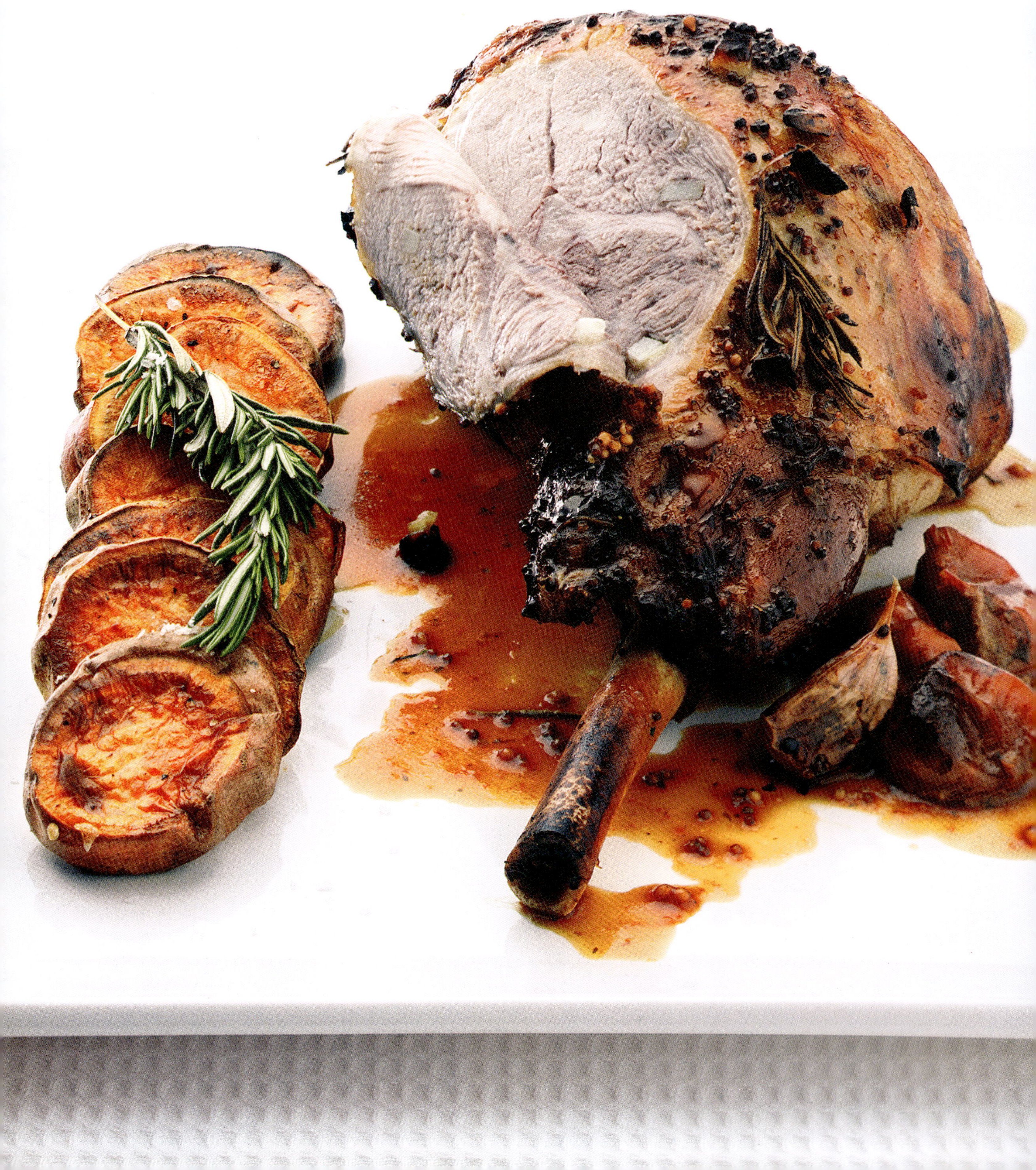

SWEET ROAST LAMB

(opposite)

This is a good, high-protein meal. Leftovers can be eaten cold with salad, or reheated the next day.

1 leg of lamb
3 cloves garlic, sliced lengthways
4 tablespoons tamari
2 teaspoons coarse-grain mustard
2 teaspoons honey
fresh rosemary
1 bulb garlic
12–15 cherry tomatoes, preferably on the vine

Preheat the oven to 375°F/gas mark 5. Wash the lamb and trim off any excess fat. Make incisions into the meat with a sharp knife and push slices of garlic into the slits. For the sauce, mix the tamari, mustard, and honey in a mug and top up with boiling water.

Lay the lamb in a roasting pan on top of some of the rosemary and pour the sauce all over it. Place the garlic bulb beside the lamb. Arrange the cherry tomatoes around the meat. The tomatoes will gradually turn mushy, but they add to the flavor of the gravy. Top with the rest of the fresh rosemary. Roast in the oven, basting every 20 minutes. Allow a cooking time of 25 minutes per pound (55 minutes per kilogram). Add another ½–1 cup of boiling water to the bottom of the roasting pan half way through cooking to make a rich gravy.

Serve with freshly steamed broccoli or other green vegetables and roasted sweet potatoes.

Serves 4

GOBBLE PIE

This is a healthier version of a traditional meat-and-potato pie. A vegetarian version of this dish can be made using 2 7-oz (200-g) cans of fava or other beans instead of turkey.

1 lb (500 g) potatoes
1 large onion, chopped
2 cloves garlic, crushed
1 tablespoon olive oil
2 tablespoons water
1 carrot, finely chopped
1 stick celery, finely chopped
1 lb (500 g) turkey mince
¾ cup (200 g) canned tomatoes
2 tablespoons chopped parsley
2 teaspoons tamari or soy sauce
2 teaspoons Worcestershire sauce
1 bay leaf
1 tablespoon olive oil
1 tablespoon sesame seeds

Peel the potatoes, put them in a pan of cold water and bring to the boil. Meanwhile, soften the onion and garlic in the tablespoon of olive oil and 2 tablespoons of water. Add the carrot, celery, and turkey mince and stir until the meat is browned. Add the tomatoes, parsley, tamari or soy sauce, Worcestershire sauce, and bay leaf and stir well. Cover and leave to simmer. Check every now and then, and add water if it is drying out. Preheat the oven to 400°F/gas mark 6.

Meanwhile, when the potatoes are cooked, drain and mash them with 1 tablespoon of olive oil and season. Remove the bay leaf from the mince and put the meat in an ovenproof casserole dish, keeping back some of the liquid if it is very watery. Season with freshly ground black pepper. Top the meat with the mashed potatoes and sprinkle the sesame seeds on top. Bake for 20–30 minutes, or until the potato is golden brown. Serve with steamed broccoli.

Serves 4

SEATOWN KEDGEREE

I love this version of a so-called kedgeree because I'm not a fan of cold, hard-cooked eggs with fish. But, you could add eggs if you like.

½ cup (100 g) brown rice
1 onion, finely diced
handful of seedless white raisins
splash of olive oil
knob of butter
2 smoked-mackerel fillets
handful of sunflower seeds

Put the rice on to boil. Gently cook the onion and raisins in the olive oil and butter—be careful not to let them brown much. Remove the skin from the mackerel fillets and break the fish up. When the rice is cooked, fold all the ingredients in together and sprinkle sunflower seeds over the top. Serve with a fresh spinach salad.

Serves 2

BARBEQUED SQUID

This is another great seafood recipe from my friend James Verner. The squid should be so fresh that the suckers stick to your fingers. (You can replace the chili sherry with ordinary sherry mixed with a finely chopped chili.)

½ lb (250 g) squid
½ onion
½ red pepper
extra-virgin olive oil
chili sherry (see below)
sea salt
½ lemon

If the fish seller hasn't already done so, first clean the squid, removing the ink sac, skin, and fins. Cut into rings, but leave the head and tentacles intact.

Cut the pepper and onion into slices about the same size as the squid rings—there should be roughly the same number of pieces of onion and pepper as of squid. Thread the pieces onto 4 sharp skewers, alternating squid, pepper, and onion. The squid head goes on last (secured on the skewer with the 2 fins); wrap the tentacles back around each skewer. Place the skewers in a tray and drizzle over some olive oil and then the chili sherry. Leave to marinate for about an hour, basting occasionally.

Sear on a fierce heat for no more than a minute. Before removing from flame, pour on the juice from the tray. Sprinkle with salt, squeeze the half lemon over the skewers, and serve.
Serves 4

For the chili sherry:
2 cups (500 ml) Amontillado
1 fresh, red chili

Put the chili in a dark bottle. Add the sherry. Leave for one year and then handle with care.

SHIITAKE ROAST CHICKEN

The secret to this recipe is the gravy in which the chicken cooks, and the use of an organic chicken. If you buy a larger bird and cook it accordingly, the leftovers make for a great salad the next day. If you are not a big fan of mushrooms, you can always leave out the shiitake, although they do have an amazing taste and texture and are very good for your immune system.

3 lb (1½ kg) organic chicken
4–6 cloves garlic, sliced lengthways
2–3 whole cloves garlic
4 tablespoons tamari
1 lemon
8–12 dried shiitake mushrooms
freshly ground black pepper
2 teaspoons honey
1 cup boiling water

Preheat the oven to 375°F/gas mark 5. Wash the chicken, dry it with paper towels, and put it in a roasting pan. Use a sharp knife to make incisions in the breasts and fleshy legs of the chicken and insert slices of garlic into the slits. Put the whole garlic cloves in the bottom of the roasting pan. Pour in the tamari and rub it all over the bird. Cut the lemon in half and squeeze the juice all over the outside of the chicken. Then slice one of the squeezed lemon halves into three and lay the pieces over the top of the chicken. Place the other lemon half inside the cavity. Arrange the shiitake mushrooms around the chicken and grind black pepper all over it. Add the honey to a mug of boiling water and stir well so that it dissolves completely. Pour this mixture into the bottom of the roasting pan.

Roast the chicken in the oven for about 1 hour, 15 minutes, or until the juices between the leg and the body run clear when tested with a sharp knife. Baste the meat every 20 minutes during cooking.

Serve with steamed green vegetables and Roasted Sweet Vegetables (see page 117).
Serves 4

LENTILS WITH SPINACH

(opposite)

This Irani dish was traditionally prepared in medieval times to heal the sick. However, it was said that the dish only acted as an effective cure if the ingredients were bought with money begged in the streets.

1 cup (250 g) brown lentils
1 lb (500 g) fresh spinach or ½ lb (250 g) frozen spinach
½ teaspoon ground coriander
½ teaspoon ground cumin
1 clove garlic, crushed
freshly ground black pepper

pinch of salt
1 tablespoon olive oil

Put the lentils in a pan of cold water, bring to the boil and then simmer until they are soft—this should take about an hour. Wash and chop the fresh spinach (or defrost if you're using frozen). Put the spices, garlic, pepper, salt, and olive oil in a pan over a medium heat. Stir well for a minute before adding the spinach. Stir for a couple more minutes. Drain the lentils, combine with the spinach and serve. Serves 4

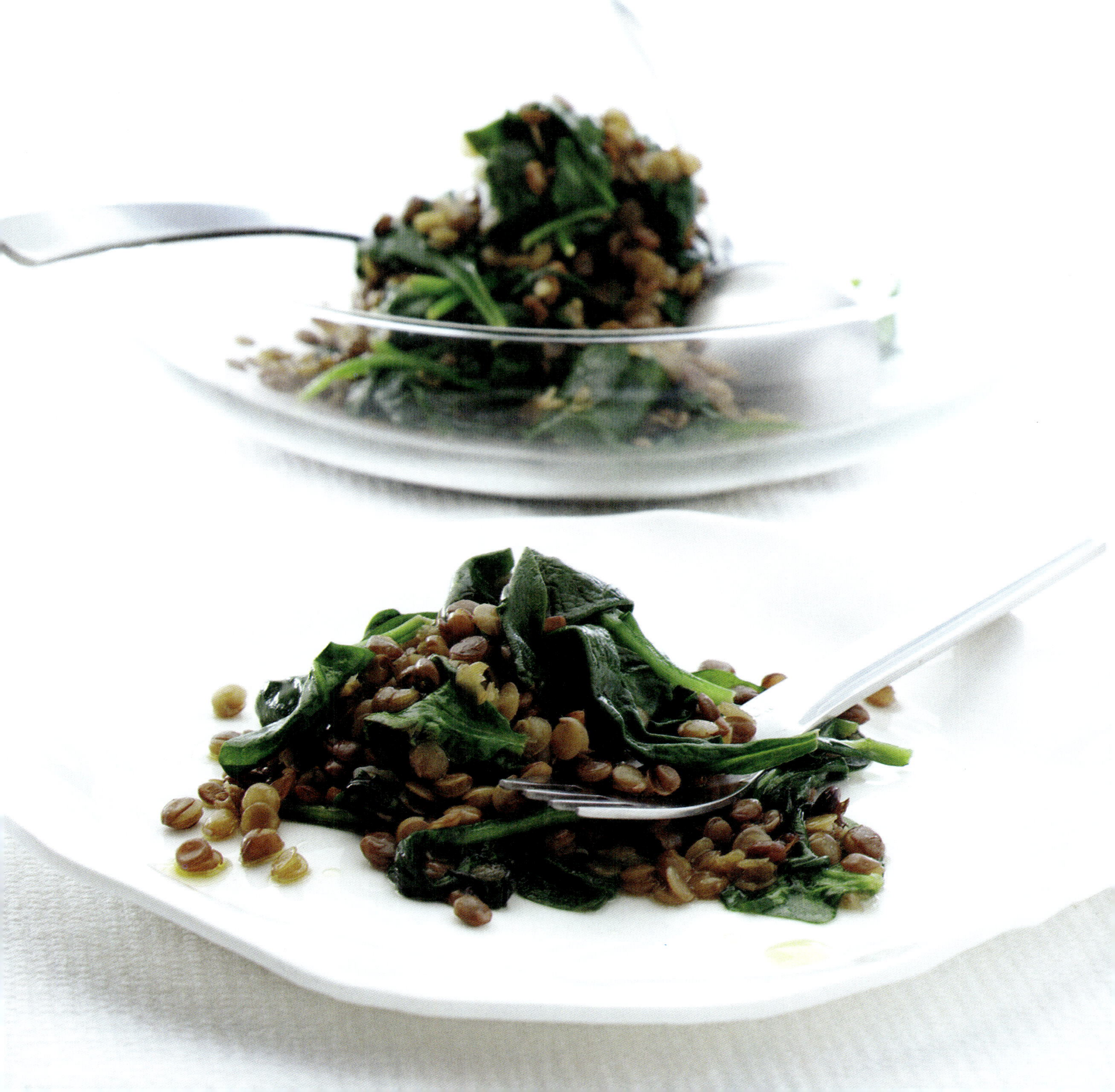

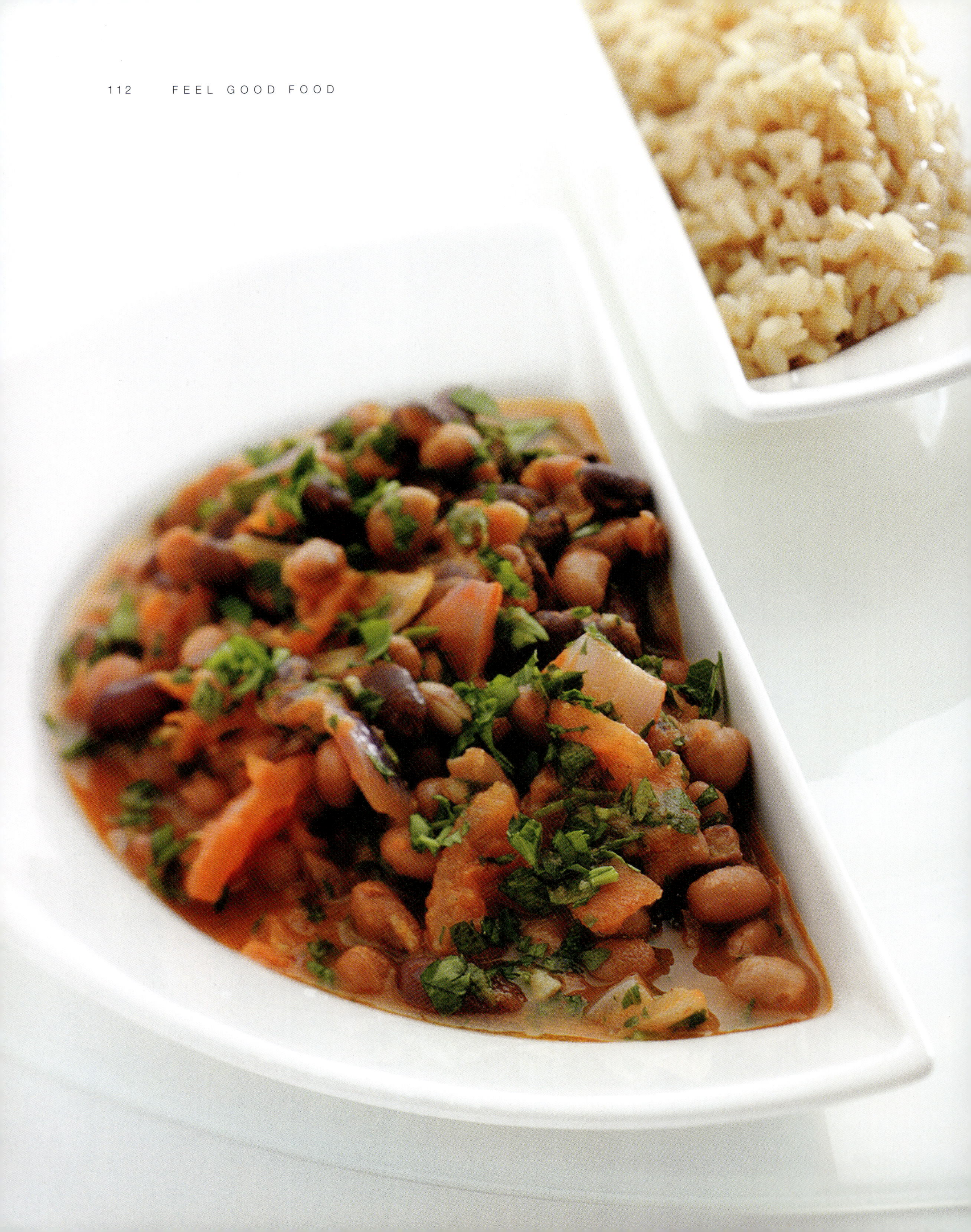

SPICED BEAN STEW

(opposite)

Although this dish is nothing like anything I ate as a child, I just love the mixture of spices. The richness of the Arabic-style cuisine conjures up images not only of the meals I used to enjoy in the Middle East but also on my travels in East Africa. If you like, you can spice the beans up further by adding a dash of chili powder.

1 onion, peeled and chopped
2 cloves garlic, peeled and crushed
½ tablespoon olive oil
1 teaspoon ground cumin
½ teaspoon ground cardamom
½ teaspoon paprika
½ teaspoon ground cinnamon
3 large tomatoes, peeled and chopped
2 lb (420-g) cans mixed beans, drained
1 empty bean can water
parsley to garnish

Soften the onions and garlic in a large pan with the olive oil. Add the powdered spices and stir well for a few minutes. Add in the tomatoes and then the beans. Pour in a can of water and leave the mixture to simmer for at least half an hour until stewed.

Serve the stew garnished with a generous amount of chopped parsley and accompanied by brown rice.

Serves 3–4

QUINOA WITH ROAST VEGETABLES

This is my variation on a dish that is usually made with cous cous. Quinoa is unusually high in protein for a grain.

1 red pepper
1 green pepper
2 red onions
2 zucchini
2 large Portobello mushrooms
8–10 cherry tomatoes
8–10 cloves garlic
olive oil
a few sprigs of fresh thyme
freshly ground black pepper
sea salt
1 cup quinoa
2 cups water

Wash and slice all the vegetables except the tomatoes and garlic (cut the onion into no more than 4 pieces). Leave the tomatoes whole and the garlic cloves in their skins. Toss all the vegetables together in a large roasting tin with plenty of olive oil and the thyme. Season with freshly ground black pepper and a little sea salt.

Roast at 350°F/gas mark 4 for 30–40 minutes, or until all the vegetables are soft and turning brown at the edges.

Meanwhile, rinse the quinoa thoroughly and put it in a saucepan with the water. (If quinoa is not rinsed well, it can be a bit bitter.) Bring to the boil, then cover and turn down to simmer until it is cooked. This should take about 15 minutes.

Serve a mound of quinoa topped with a selection of the vegetables and drizzled with a little olive oil.

Serves 4

SHEKSHOUKA

This refreshing Maltese dish has its roots in Tunisia. My grandmother used to serve it as a meal in itself, dropping in a couple of fresh eggs at the last minute and cooking until they had set. I leave them out, as I don't like peppers mixed with eggs. You can also serve Shekshouka as a side dish to accompany meat or fish.

8 small tomatoes
2 medium-sized green peppers
2 medium-sized onions
2 teaspoons extra-virgin olive oil
3 tablespoons water
freshly ground black pepper
pinch of salt

Put the tomatoes in a bowl and pour boiling water over them. Core, deseed, and slice the peppers and then peel and slice the onions. Gently take the tomatoes out of the water with a spoon, then peel, deseed, and cut them into quarters. Soften the peppers and onions in the heated olive oil and water. Season with salt and pepper.

When the peppers have softened, add the tomato quarters until they, too, are soft.

Serve on a mound of steaming brown rice or quinoa.

Serves 3–4

side dishes, side salads

PROPER GREEN SALAD

(main image, opposite)

If you're put off a green salad because it conjures up unpleasant images of insipid iceberg lettuce and a few slices of cucumber, think again. This is a side dish brimming with textures and flavors. And, of course, the dressing makes all the difference.

2 generous handfuls baby spinach
4 florets broccoli, trimmed
2 tablespoons white cabbage, shredded
1 handful watercress
1 handful sprouted alfalfa
1 handful sprouted mung beans
2 inches (5 cm) cucumber, diced
1 tablespoon pumpkin seeds

Toss all the ingredients together in a large bowl and serve with one of the salad dressings. If you think there may be any leftovers, dress the salad on individual plates rather than in the large serving bowl.
Serves 4

SALAD DRESSINGS

With a great dressing, even the humblest of salad vegetables can be taken out of the refrigerator and quickly turned into a feast. The best way to make these dressings is to put the ingredients in a jar and shake them well. They will keep in the refrigerator for about a week.

Creamy Vinaigrette

6 tablespoons olive oil
2 tablespoons balsamic vinegar
1 heaped teaspoon coarsegrain mustard
freshly ground black pepper

Tangy Vinaigrette

6 tablespoons olive oil
2 tablespoons lemon juice
1 heaped teaspoon smooth green-peppercorn mustard
1 clove garlic, crushed
pinch of salt

Oriental Bite

3 tablespoons olive oil
2 teaspoons sesame oil
juice of 2 limes
2 teaspoons chopped coriander
3 dashes Tobasco sauce

Rich Pesto Dressing

1 teaspoon pesto
4 tablespoons olive oil
juice of ½ lemon
freshly ground black pepper
pinch salt

TABOULEH *(top inset image, right)*

This is a variation on the traditional Lebanese Tabouleh, using quinoa instead of bulgur wheat. It makes a great accompaniment to broiled meat.

3 level tablespoons quinoa
6 tablespoons water
1 large bunch parsley, finely chopped
3 stalks fresh mint, finely chopped
3 scallions, finely sliced
3 medium-sized tomatoes, roughly chopped
3 tablespoons olive oil
1 tablespoon fresh lemon juice
pinch sea salt
1 tomato, sliced
lettuce leaves

Rinse the quinoa thoroughly—if it is not rinsed well, it can be bitter. Put it in a saucepan with the water. Bring to the boil, cover, and then simmer until cooked (about 15 minutes). Leave to cool. Mix the quinoa with the chopped parsley, mint, scallions, tomatoes, olive oil, lemon juice, and salt. Taste to see if you may prefer it a bit more lemony. Arrange on a large serving plate surrounded by crisp lettuce leaves. Garnish with slices of tomato.
Serves 2–3

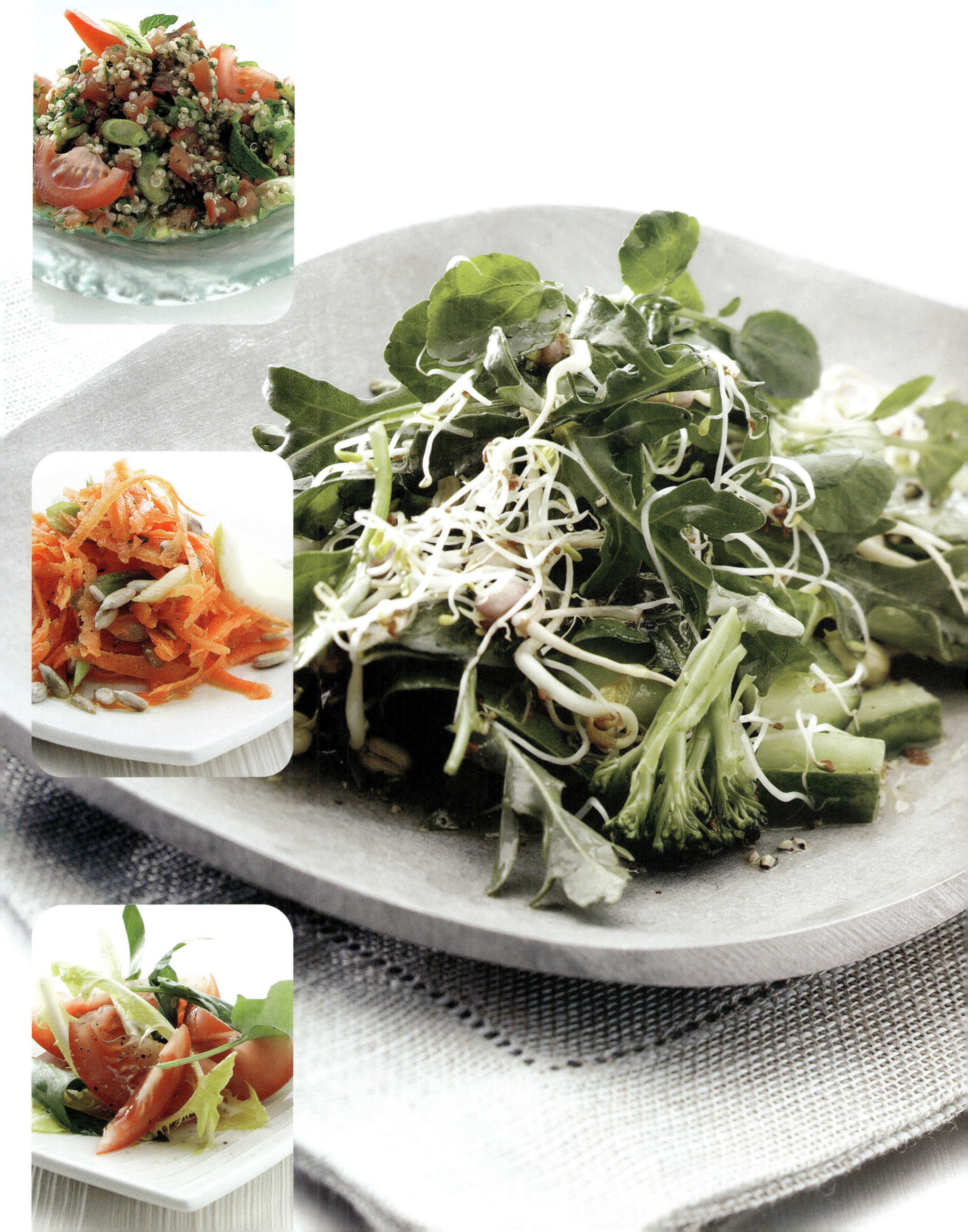

CRUNCHY ORIENTAL SALAD

I could eat this wonderful salad every day. The shredded cabbage makes it truly crunchy.

palmful of dried seaweed, such as arame
2 medium-sized carrots
¼ white cabbage, shredded
3 scallions, finely sliced
fresh coriander—about 10 stalks, roughly chopped
2 teaspoons sesame oil
juice of 2 limes
1 tablespoon tamari or soy sauce
1 tablespoon sesame seeds

Put the seaweed in a mug, pour on just about enough boiling water to cover, and leave to steep. Meanwhile, grate the carrots into a large bowl, adding the white cabbage, scallion, and coriander. Check the seaweed is soft and drain in a sieve, tossing it to allow it to cool off before adding it to the salad. Add the sesame oil, lime juice, and tamari, and toss all the ingredients together well.

Just before serving, sprinkle with the sesame seeds.

Serves 3

CRUNCHY CARROT SALAD *(below)*

Sometimes I just have a big bowl of this and a couple of hard-cooked eggs for lunch. You can make the salad even crunchier by adding some shredded cabbage.

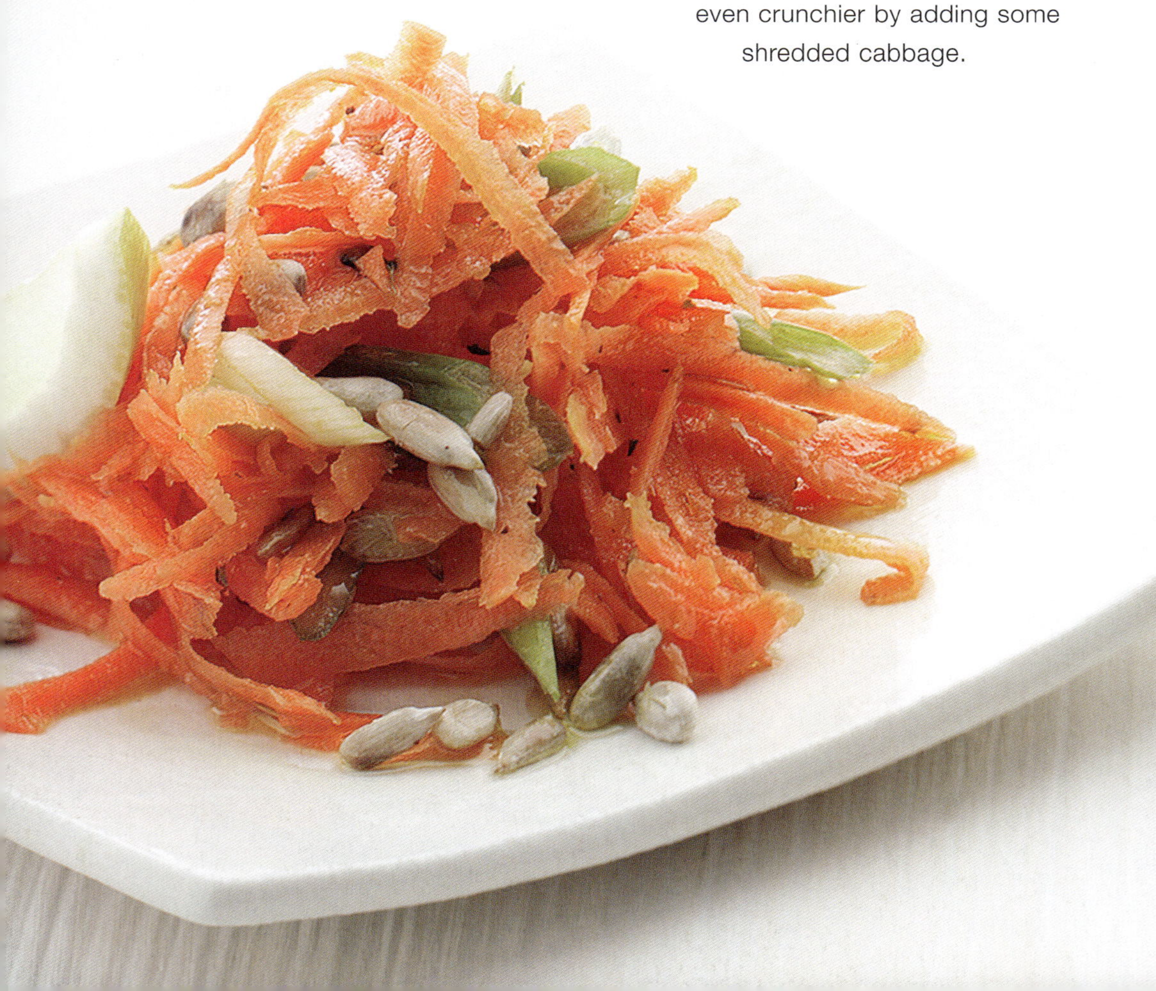

3 medium-sized carrots
3 scallions, finely sliced
1 tablespoon olive oil
juice of ½ lemon
1 tablespoon toasted sunflower seeds

Grate the carrots and toss together with all the other ingredients.

Serves 2

SOM TAM

Traditionally from the Isaan region of northeastern Thailand, this dish is made freshly to order with a mortar and pestle at street stalls and served with sticky rice and broiled chicken. This is a *som tam farang*—foreigner's *som tam*—minus the copious chilies, pungent dried shrimps, and whole, pickled, raw crab! It's best to visit your local Asian grocers to stock up on the ingredients. If you cannot get hold of green papaya, use half a white cabbage instead. Also, the cashews are actually supposed to be peanuts.

½ green papaya, finely shredded
4 cherry tomatoes
10 scarlet runner beans
2 tablespoons roasted cashew nuts
1 clove garlic
1 bird's-eye chili
2 limes
2 teaspoons tamarind concentrate, diluted with same amount of water
1 tablespoon fish sauce
2 teaspoons coconut-palm sugar (*jageree* from Indian grocers)

In a mortar, crush the garlic, chili, coconut-palm sugar, and cashew nuts. Add the beans and tomato, pounding all the time.

Little by little, add the shredded papaya, pounding all the time. Slowly add the juice of the limes, the tamarind juice, and fish sauce, continuing to pound. Taste to see whether you prefer it a little sharper (with a little more lime and tamarind) or saltier (with a little more fish sauce). Serve immediately.

Serves 4

WILD TOMATO SALAD

(below, right)

Another delicious recipe from my friend James Verner, who walks out of the door of his home in Dorset, in England, to find some of his best ingredients growing wild.

6 wild-sorrel leaves
6 stalks wild garlic
2 tomatoes
4 dandelion leaves
2 teaspoons extra-virgin olive oil
juice of 1 lemon
sea salt
freshly ground black pepper

Pick the wild leaves and garlic, rinse and cut coarsely. Cut the tomatoes into quarters or eighths. Toss the whole lot in a bowl with oil and lemon juice (even add a little zest!). Sprinkle the salad with salt and pepper. Eat immediately.

Serves 2

ROASTED SWEET VEGETABLES

I developed a taste for sweet potatoes and butternut living in Sydney, where they are a standard accompaniment to any roast dinner. They make a good starch part of any meal, even a hastily prepared supper, as they cook relatively quickly. When you are buying sweet potatoes, go for the ones with the orange flesh, rather than the white, as they are sweeter. You can always make double quantities depending on how many other vegetables you are serving with the roast or to have left-overs for lunch the next day, which you can eat cold with a salad.

1 large sweet potato
½ butternut squash
2 fresh beets
freshly ground black pepper
extra-virgin olive oil

Preheat the oven to 375°F/gas mark 5. Scrub the potatoes and slice into rounds that are each about ½ inch (1¼ cm) thick. Wash the butternut and, using a large, sharp knife, slice it, leaving the skin on. Scrub, top, and tail the beets and cut into ½-inch (1¼-cm) slices. Place the vegetables on a baking tray (ideally lined with baking paper to prevent them from sticking, and make washing up easier!). Drizzle olive oil all over the top and season with freshly ground black pepper.

Bake in the oven until cooked—this should take about 20–30 minutes. Prick with a skewer to check that the vegetables are soft before serving.

Serves 4

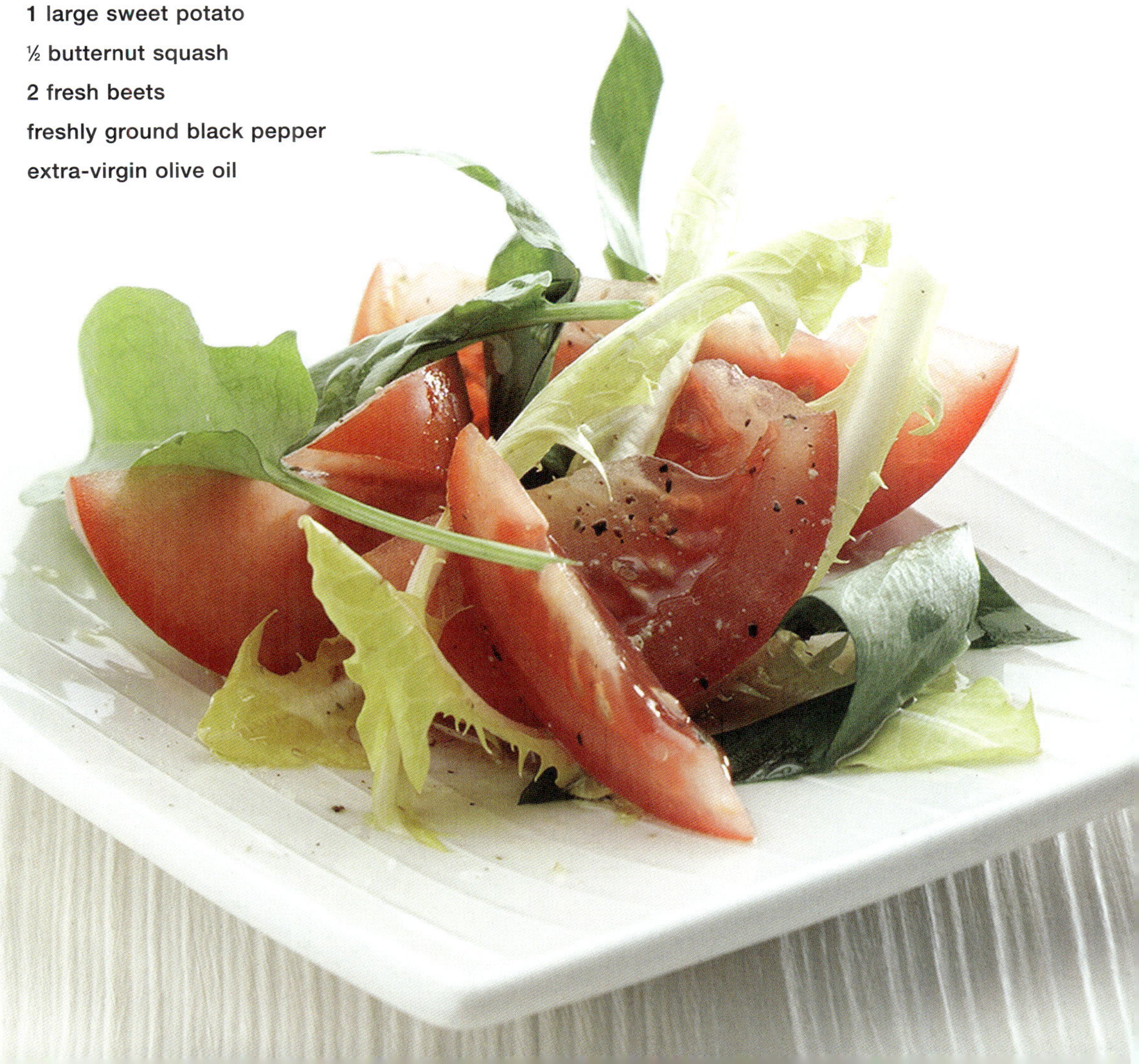

desserts

Desserts of all kinds are usually regarded as a big no-no on any sort of healthy eating program. Not so. I am not going to recommend stodgy, sugary, heavy puddings here (not that there's anything wrong with having one of those every now and then), but I will show that, with a little imagination, you can conjure up a range of delicious and healthy dishes to finish off a meal and leave your sweet taste buds feeling fully satisfied.

APRICOT ICE CREAM WITH PISTACHIOS *(main image, opposite)*

This recipe—with its subtle hint of cardamom—takes me right back to my childhood in the Middle East. Leave the cardamom out if you prefer.

3½ oz (100 g) dried apricots
5 oz (150 g) natural yogurt
½ teaspoon ground cardamom
6 tablespoons (50 g) shelled pistachio nuts
4 egg whites
4 tablespoons (50 g) fine brown sugar

Soak the apricots overnight until they are fully soft. Drain away the water and in a blender blend the apricots with the yogurt and cardamom. Put aside 8–12 whole pistachios. Crush the rest of the pistachios and add to the apricot mix. Beat the egg whites and sugar until the mixture stays in peaks. Gently fold the apricot and egg-white mixtures into one another.

Pour the mixture into a covered container and put in the freezer. Stir every 40 minutes for the first 2–3 hours to prevent ice crystals from forming. If you freeze the ice cream for longer than 3 hours, put it in the refrigerator for 20 minutes before serving. Serve topped with the whole pistachios. Serves 4

CARDAMOM FRUITS

Although the flavor of this recipe is similar to the one above because of the cardamom—a favorite of mine—it takes a lot less time and effort to make and is just as tasty.

2 cups (500 ml) water
15 cardamom pods
2 tablespoons honey
3½ oz (100 g) dried pears
3½ oz (100 g) dried peaches
3½ oz (100 g) dried apricots
juice of 1 lime
10 oz (300 g) natural yogurt
1 teaspoon honey
¼–½ teaspoon vanilla extract

Bring the water to the boil with the cardamom and honey. Turn down to simmer—after 5 minutes, add the dried fruit. Cook for 5 more minutes then add the lime juice. In a separate bowl, blend the yogurt with honey and vanilla extract. Serve the fruit hot or chilled with the vanilla yogurt. Serves 4

CHOCOLATE PUDDING

This delight is remarkably unwicked for such a luxurious result. You can vary the taste by adding a little orange juice or mint extract to give a different spin on semi-sweet chocolate.

2½ cups (600 ml) semi-skimmed milk
2½–3½ oz (75–100 g) semi-sweet, organic chocolate
4 eggs
¼ teaspoon salt
1 teaspoon vanilla extract

Put the oven on to heat up at 335°F/gas mark 3. Put the milk and chocolate in a saucepan on a low heat, stirring gently until the chocolate is melted and well mixed in with the milk. Do not allow it to boil. Remove from the heat and leave to cool.

Put the eggs, salt, and vanilla in a blender and slowly add the chocolatey milk until it is all well blended. Pour the resulting mixture into 4 oven-proof individual dishes and bake in the oven for 40 minutes.

I like this pudding hot, but you can leave it to cool, cover with plastic wrap and keep in the refrigerator until serving. Serves 4

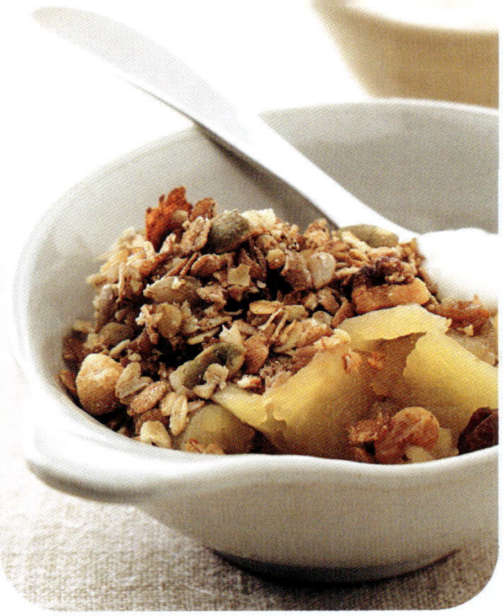
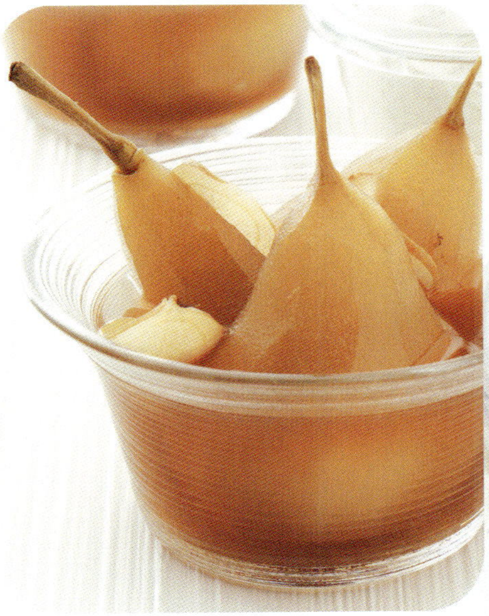
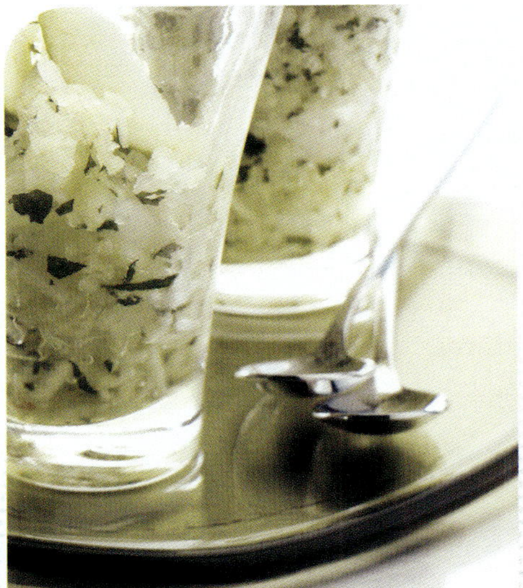
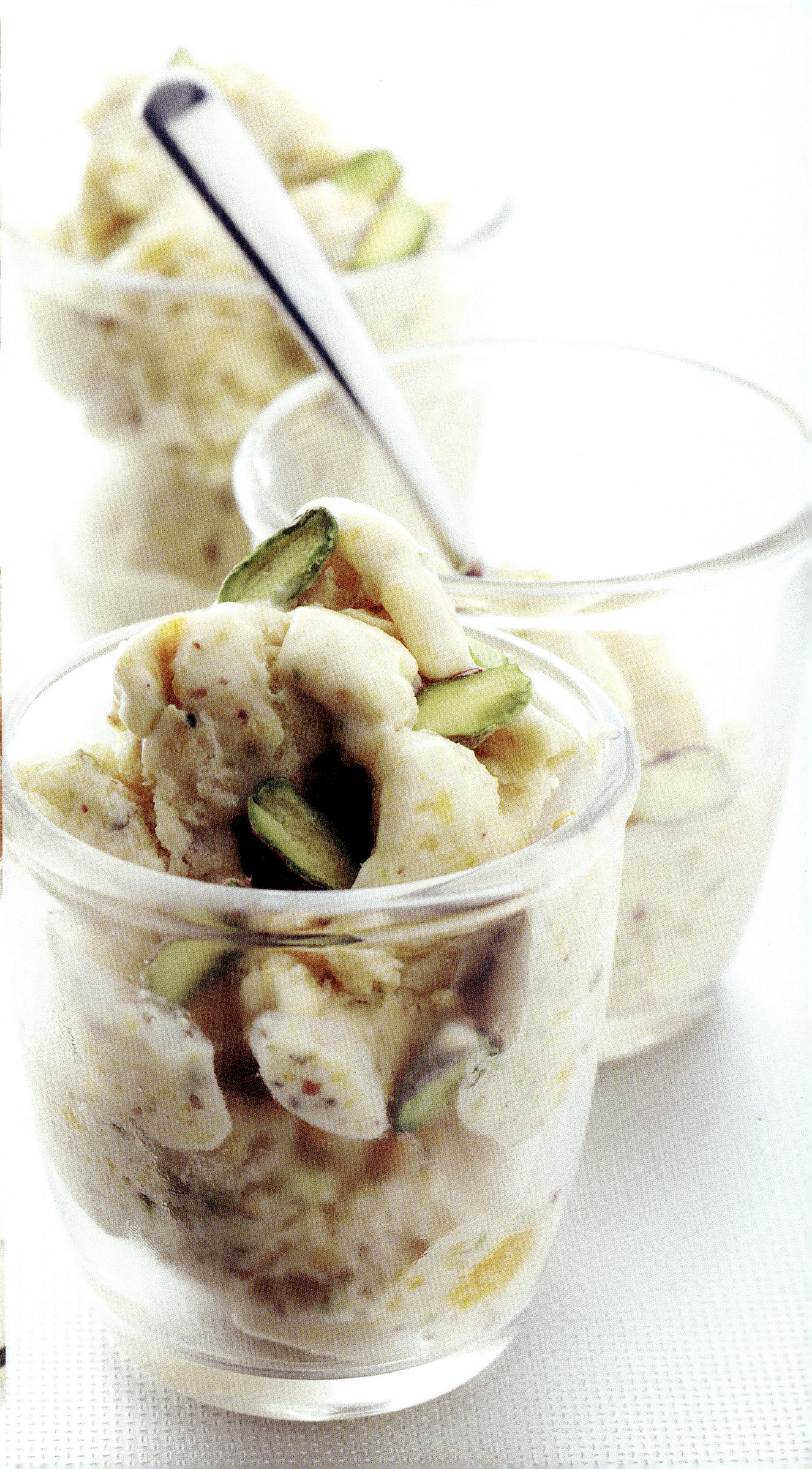

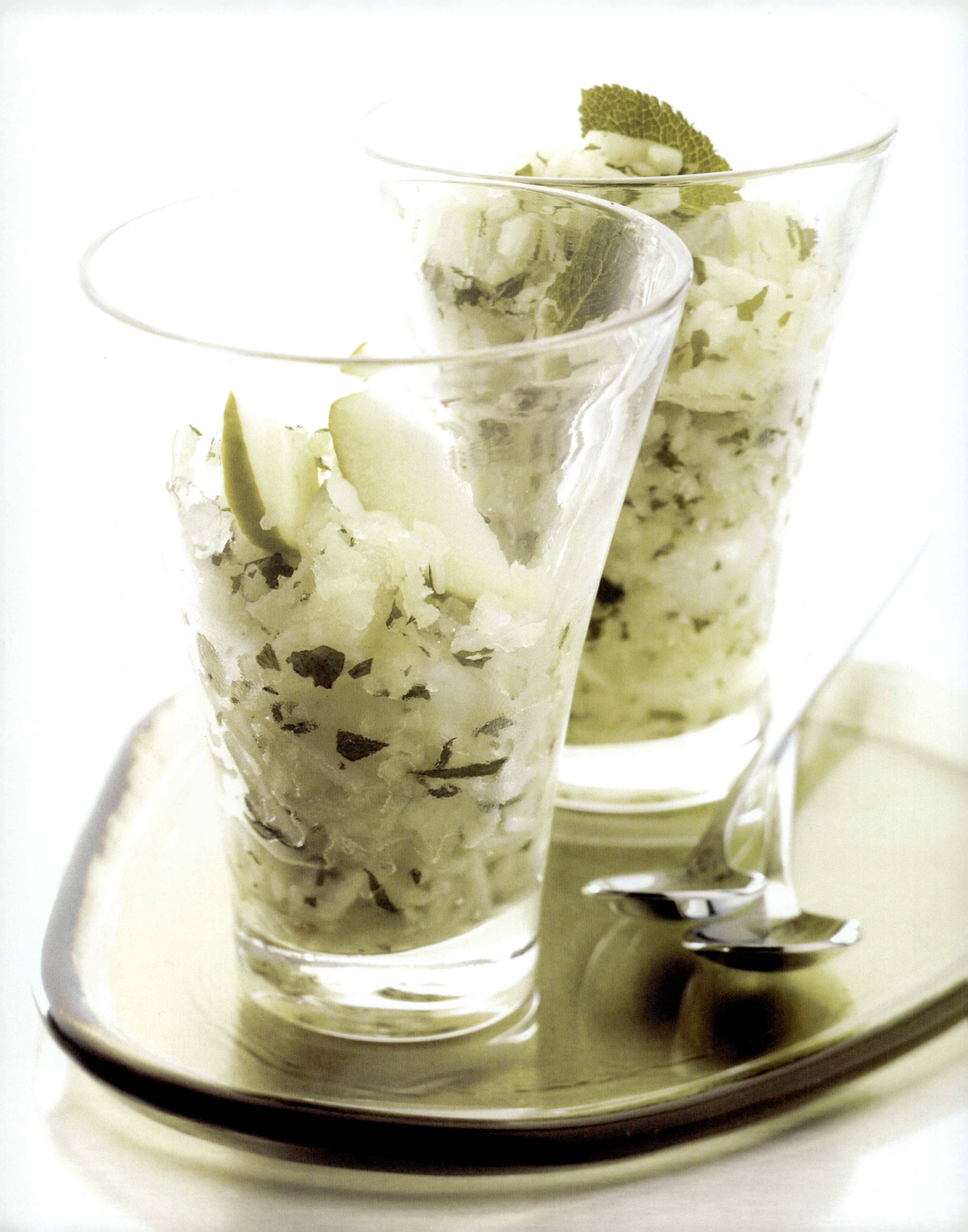

GRATED APPLE ICE

(opposite)

This makes a refreshing summer dessert or provides light relief after a heavy meal. You should be able to find the rose or orange-blossom water at a Middle Eastern grocers.

4 Granny Smith apples (or another sharp variety)
juice of 1 lemon
2 tablespoons clear honey
2 tablespoons rose or orange-blossom water
4 ice cubes
4 sprigs mint

Retain 4 thin slices of apple for the garnish. Peel and grate the rest of the apples into a glass bowl. Squeeze the lemon juice over them and stir well. Add the honey and rose or orange-blossom water and stir it all again.

Chill for at least 2 hours. Before serving, crush the ice cubes in a blender or mortar and pestle, and add to the apple mix. Roughly tear the mint leaves and stir into the apple ice. Serve garnished with the slices of apple.
Serves 4

BAKED BANANAS WITH RASPBERRY SAUCE

The sweetness of the bananas in this dish is offset sharply by the tangy raspberry sauce.

1½ cups (200 g) raspberries
grated nutmeg
2 tablespoons honey
1 tablespoon red wine
2 large bananas
juice of ½ lemon
1 tablespoon sunflower seeds
4 mint leaves

Preheat the oven to 350°F/gas mark 4. Heat the raspberries over a low heat in a pan with the nutmeg, 1 tablespoon of the honey and the wine. (Keep 4 raspberries aside for the garnish.) When the raspberries are soft, remove from the heat and process in a blender (for a rougher texture, you can also just mash them with a fork or strain them in a sieve to get rid of the seeds).

Slice the bananas in half lengthways. Put them in a dish, squeeze over the lemon juice, drizzle over 1 tablespoon of the honey, and sprinkle with sunflower seeds. Bake in the oven for 10–12 minutes.

Serve the bananas drizzled with the raspberry sauce, topped with a whole raspberry and a mint leaf.
Serves 4

CRUNCHY OATY CRUMBLE

Most people are instant converts to this version of an old favorite—there's so much texture, crunch, and flavor to it. You can replace the apples with any of your favorite fruits, or add blackberries or blackcurrants.

1 lb (500 g) muesli
2 teaspoons ground cinnamon
2 tablespoons pumpkin seeds
10 or so walnuts
⅓ stick (40 g) butter
3 large cooking apples
2 tablespoons raisins or sultanas
1 tablespoon brown sugar
4 tablespoons water

Put the muesli plus 1 teaspoon of the cinnamon powder, the pumpkin seeds, and the broken-up walnuts into a large mixing bowl with the butter, chopped into pieces. Mix with your fingers until there are no lumps of butter left. Alternatively, you can melt the butter and mix it in that way. Peel, core, and slice the apples and lay them in a baking dish, sprinkled with the raisins, remaining cinnamon, and sugar. Add 4 tablespoons of water.

Lay the crumble mixture over the top of the apples so that they are well covered. Bake in the oven at 350°F/gas mark 4 for about 40 minutes, or until the apples are soft when skewered.

Serve with vanilla yogurt (see page 118), or vanilla ice cream or custard.
Serves 4

KHOSAF

This Middle Eastern staple makes a filling dessert or a good afternoon snack. You can make this amount in advance and store it in the refrigerator to eat over a few days.

Experimenting with other dried fruits, such as figs or peaches, makes a change. You should be able to find the rose or orange-blossom water at a Middle Eastern grocers.

continued

1 tablespoon clear honey
2½ cups (300 g) dried apricots
1½ cups (250 g) prunes
½ cup (100 g) raisins
½ cup (100 g) fresh almonds
6 tablespoons (50 g) pine nuts
2 tablespoons rose or orange-blossom water (or 1 tablespoon of each)

In a large bowl, melt the honey in half a mug of boiling water. Add the fruit and nuts and cover with cold water. Pour in the rose and/or orange-blossom water and mix well. Leave in the refrigerator for at least 48 hours.

Serve the Khosaf just as it is or with the vanilla yogurt described in the Cardamom Fruits recipe on page 118.
Serves 6

FRUIT WHIZZ

These are two delicious, refreshing desserts that are super fast to make. They represent two variations on the same theme—one with summer berries and one with tropical fruits—and each has a completely different taste. The Summer Whizz, because of the hot fruit sauce, is actually lovely in the winter, too—replace the fresh summer fruits with a bag of frozen.

Summer Whizz

1 lb (500 g) fresh or frozen summer fruits
½ cup (100 g) natural yogurt
½ teaspoon vanilla extract
2 teaspoons clear honey
2 tablespoons kirsch or red wine

Place half of the fruit in a blender along with the yogurt and the vanilla extract, and blend the mixture until it is smooth.

Pour the mixture into a bowl and put it into the freezer for at least one hour. Stir it a couple of times to stop it crystallizing too much.

Meanwhile, put the rest of the fruit in a saucepan with the honey and the kirsch or wine on a low heat and gently bring to the boil for a minute or so. If it is particularly watery, simmer until the mixture reduces a bit.

Scoop the frozen whizz into bowls and pour the hot fruit sauce over the top, then serve immediately.
Serves 4

Tropical Whizz

½-lb (250-g) bag frozen tropical fruit
½ cup (100 g) natural yogurt
1 tablespoon shredded coconut
4 slices canned pineapple, in juice
2 teaspoons clear honey
2 passion fruits

Put the tropical fruit in a blender with the yogurt, coconut, and 2 tablespoons of the pineapple juice and blend it until it is completely smooth. Pour the mixture into a bowl and put it into the freezer for at least an hour. Stir it a couple of times to stop it crystallizing too much.

Meanwhile, drizzle the honey over the pineapple slices and put them into a heated griddle pan for 1–2 minutes on each side until they start to turn slightly brown.

Put a pineapple slice on each plate and top with a scoop of the whizz. Slice the passion fruits in half and scoop the contents of each half on top of the whizz. Serve immediately.
Serves 4

FIRESIDE PEARS *(opposite)*

I first made this to eat around a woodburning stove on a winter's night in Dorset, England, and it's been a warming favorite ever since. If you like cloves, try adding a few when you make the ginger sauce.

2 cups (500 ml) water
1½ tablespoons soft brown sugar
½ inch (1¼ cm) gingerroot, finely sliced
2 tablespoons of kirsch
4 firm pears
6 tablespoons crème fraîche
¼ teaspoon cinnamon powder
4 mint leaves

Put the water, sugar, and ginger in a saucepan and bring to the boil before adding the kirsch. Leave to simmer for 10 minutes.

Meanwhile, peel the pears, cut them in half and lay them in an oven-proof dish. Pour the ginger sauce over the pears and bake in the oven at 350°F/ gas mark 4 for 30 minutes.

Mix the crème fraîche with the cinnamon. When the pears are tender, serve two halves in each bowl. Place a dollop of the crème fraîche on top or serve it in a small bowl on the side. Garnish each pear half with a mint leaf.
Serves 4

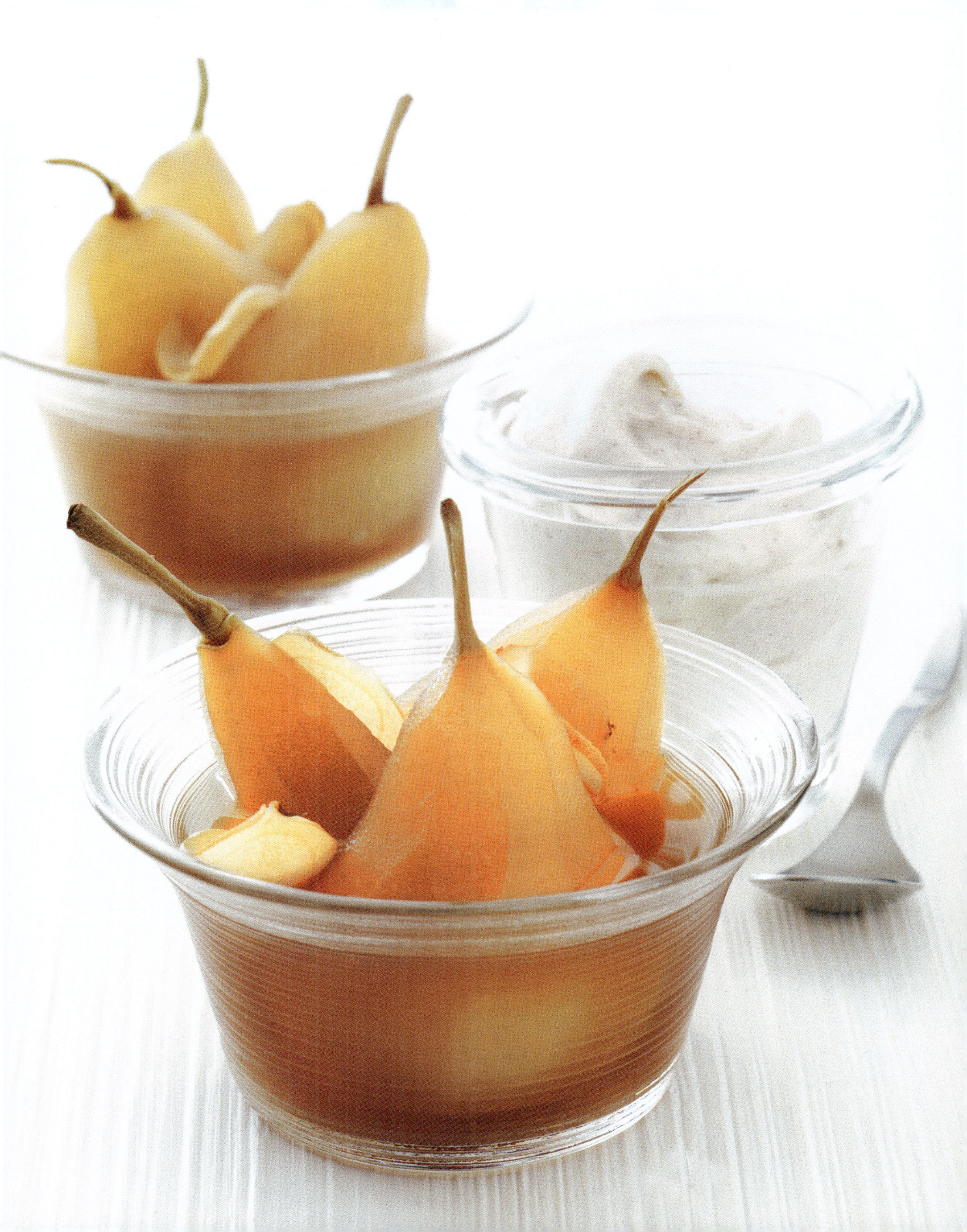

snacks

Grazing, or having a little snack in between meals, is no bad thing. For many of us, it is actually the best way to eat as far as balancing our blood sugar is concerned. This is largely because if we wait too long from one meal to the next, blood-sugar levels take a dive and with them our energy, mood, and concentration.

Snacks that release energy fast—such as something very sweet or a coffee—may well do the trick of getting you out of a trough quickly, but you're likely to need to grab another snack soon afterward. Slow-releasing snacks—that gradually and evenly raise your blood-sugar levels—are much better for you. Obviously, this whole mechanism depends on your metabolism and what your last meal was (see pages 12–17), but you can avoid a slump by having a satisfying, healthy snack.

FRESH FRUIT WITH NATURAL YOGURT

Choose berries and cherries in the summer, juicy ripe pears and a variety of apples in the winter, or any fruit you fancy. A couple of exceptions—don't keep resorting to bananas, which are very sweet and fast-releasing.

Accompanied by a small pot or a couple of tablespoons of natural yogurt, fruit makes a satisfying mini-meal. You could have a few pieces of dried fruit, but remember they are a very concentrated form of sugar and should be eaten in only small amounts. Also, some people find dried fruit makes them bloated.

FRESH NUTS AND SEEDS

Go for fresh almonds, filberts, cashews, or Brazils, and avoid nuts that are roasted or salted. For seeds, have a mixture of pumpkin, sunflower, and sesame. Chew them all well to get the most out of their goodness. You may find it easier, and more varied, to pour a bag of each into a large container and take out a handful, or if you're out or on the go, a small bagful.

FRESH FRUIT WITH NUTS OR SEEDS

Instead of yogurt, have a handful of mixed nuts and/or seeds with your fruit. You can also make Khosaf (see page 121) as a good teatime snack.

RAW CARROTS AND OTHER VEGETABLES

Crudités, or raw vegetables, are a very refreshing between-meal snack, especially dipped in a little houmous or cottage cheese. Go for a variety, such as carrots, broccoli, cauliflower, celery, or radishes. Most supermarkets sell ready-washed and cut bagfuls of these vegetables—they're a good snack to pick up on the run.

CRACKERS WITH TOPPINGS

Choose from oat cakes, rice cakes, or rye crackers and top them with:

- **houmous, goat's cheese, or cottage cheese with tomatoes, alfalfa sprouts, or radishes**
- **filbert or almond butter (you can buy all sorts of tasty nut butters from healthfood stores)**
- **smoked-fish pâté (see page 87)**

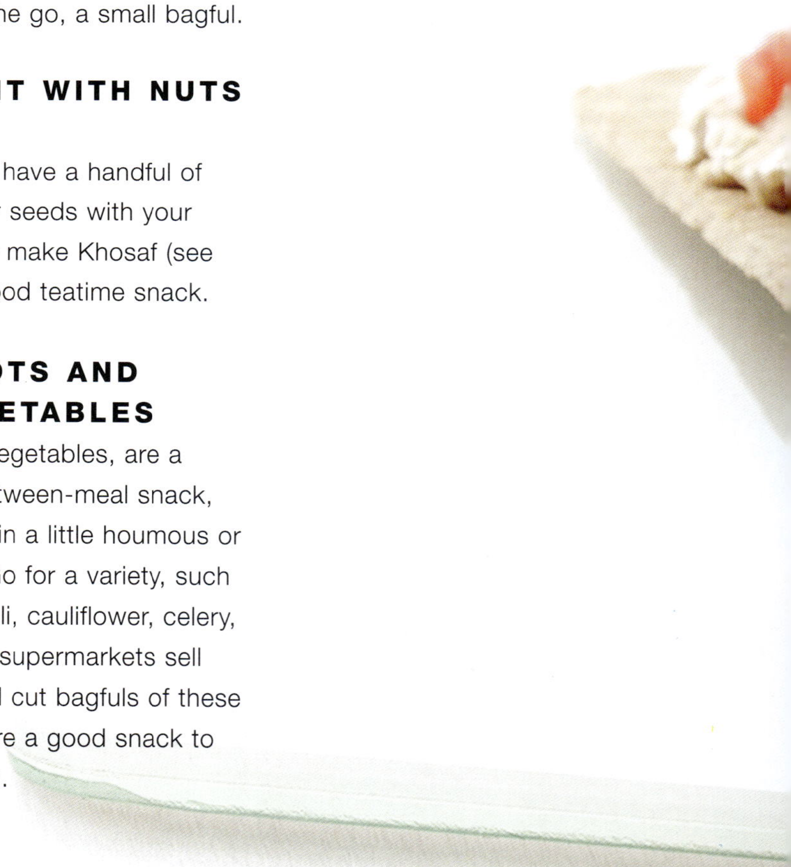

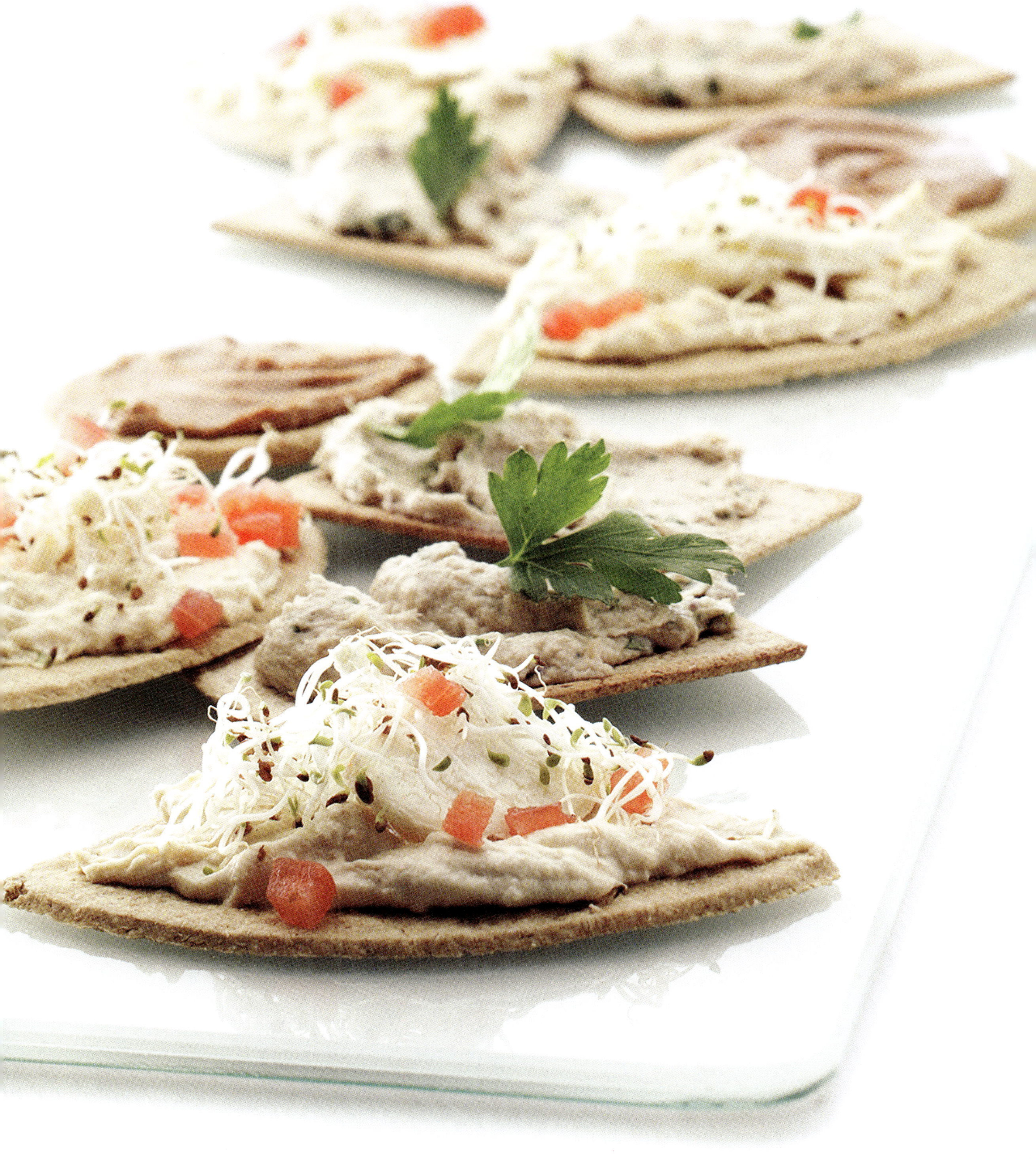

GOOD NUTRITION FORMS JUST ONE PART OF THE MIND–BODY CANVAS, AND DIETARY IMPROVEMENTS ALONE ARE NOT ALWAYS ENOUGH TO OVERCOME ON-GOING LOW MOODS. IN THIS CHAPTER WE EXPLORE A RANGE OF STRATEGIES TO COMPLEMENT A BALANCED DIET AND HELP TO KEEP YOU IN PEAK PHYSICAL AND EMOTIONAL HEALTH.

As well as eating a good diet based on the advice given in chapters 1, 2, and 3, you could consider taking nutritional supplements—these optimize your nutritional status and can dramatically enhance how you feel. However, to complete the picture of good health and to maintain even moods, it is also essential that you make other positive lifestyle changes. Doing regular, gentle exercise, sharing your problems and inner feelings with someone else (whether that person is a friend or a professional), and being aware of your approach to major life events can provide you with the sense of equilibrium that is essential for a joyful, fulfilling existence.

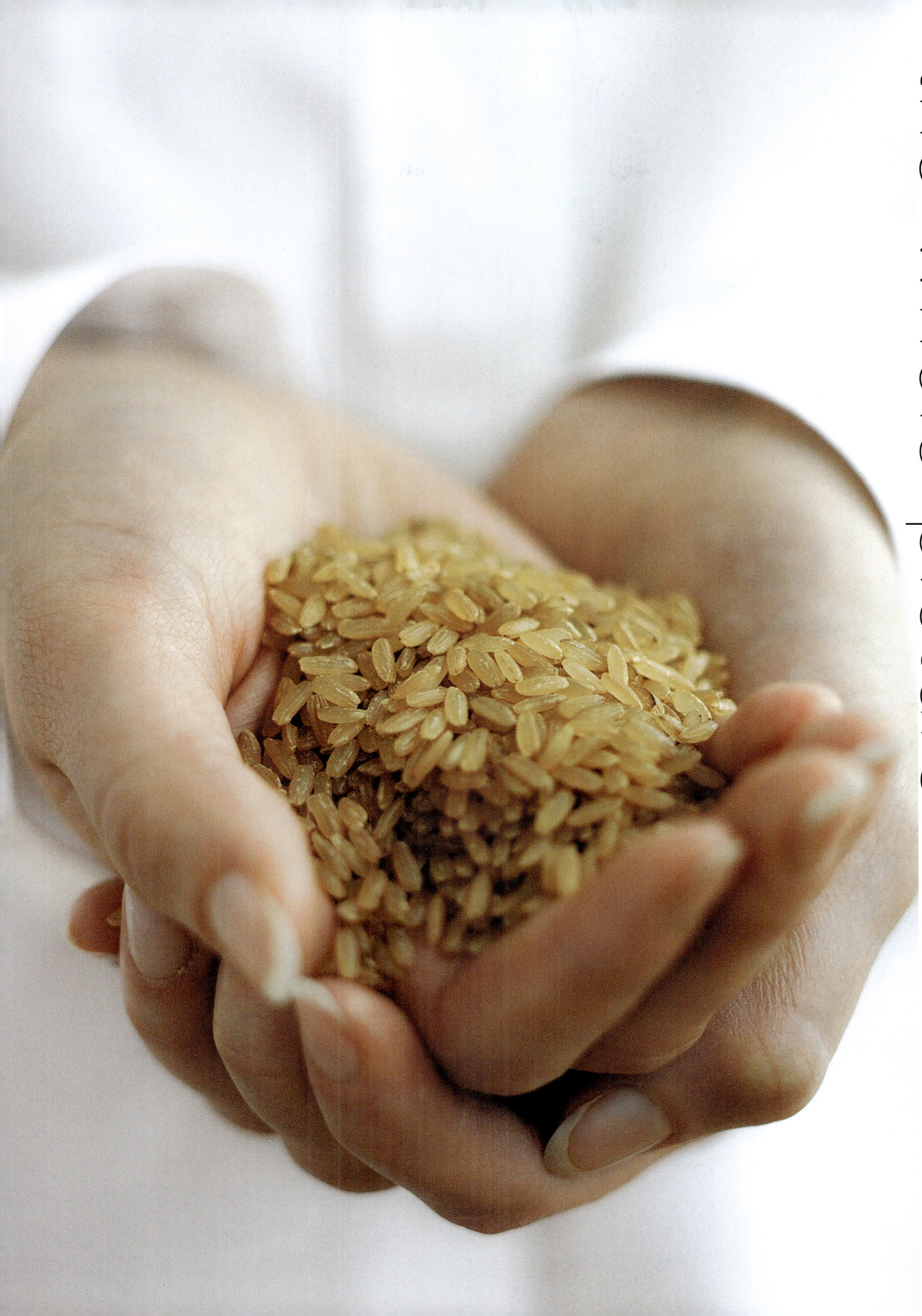

the whole picture

Taking nutritional supplements that are right for you can boost your energy and mood, minimize your risk of getting ill, and generally help you look and feel better. However, supplements should not replace a healthy, balanced diet, and are best taken with professional guidance.

feel good supplements

Positive as nutritional supplements can be, we must not forget what they are. It may seem obvious but, as their name suggests, they are meant to supplement a good diet—they are not a substitute for one. It's all too easy to cut corners with our diets, mistakenly hoping for magic-bullet-style compensation from popping pills. Unfortunately, feeling good doesn't come as simply or mechanically as that.

Whether we actually need to take supplements at all is a subject of much debate. Traditionalists may argue that we can get all the nutrients we need from a good diet. Indeed, a varied, balanced, healthy diet consisting of chemical-free, fresh food and void of substances that drain nutrients, such as alcohol and sweet sodas, would probably provide an optimum nutrient intake. However, very few of us manage consistently to eat that well. Some of the opponents of food supplements may claim that there has been too little research into their use, particularly at high doses. In some cases this may be a valid argument, although a great deal more scientific research has been done into the benefits and safety of natural nutrients than many may realize.

If you do choose to take supplements, deciding which are best for you can in itself be a minefield. Your local health store or pharmacy probably stocks countless supplements, each claiming purported benefits and a wide range of qualities. Although we all have different individual nutritional requirements, a basic program can make a great difference to how you feel. The best place to start is with a good, all-round, multi-supplement to cover all bases: one that contains all the vitamins, most minerals, and perhaps even a few extras, such as plant extracts with antioxidant or cleansing properties. When choosing a multi-supplement, bear in mind that, as with most things in life, you usually get what you pay for, so cutting costs can sometimes be a false economy. Other than basic multi-supplements, any food supplements are best taken under the guidance of a qualified nutritionist or other healthcare professional. If you are pregnant or on medication, it is essential that you seek advice from your doctor.

Controversy also surrounds the issue of supplement dosage. There are often large discrepancies between governments' recommended daily intakes and those recommended by some healthcare practitioners. This gap is, in part, owing to the fact that most standard government recommendations are based on the amount of a nutrient required to prevent symptoms of a deficiency. However, research and practice usually show that much higher levels are required for optimum health. As long as you follow the recommendations given by your healthcare practitioner or printed on the bottle of a supplement, you are unlikely to experience any adverse effects.

The ideal is to have a personal supplements program designed by a qualified nutritionist. Nevertheless, you can make a tremendous difference by following the general recommendations in this book, even without your own tailored program. However, if you would like to tackle a variety of nutritional imbalances, it is best to do this with the help of a healthcare professional (see page 139).

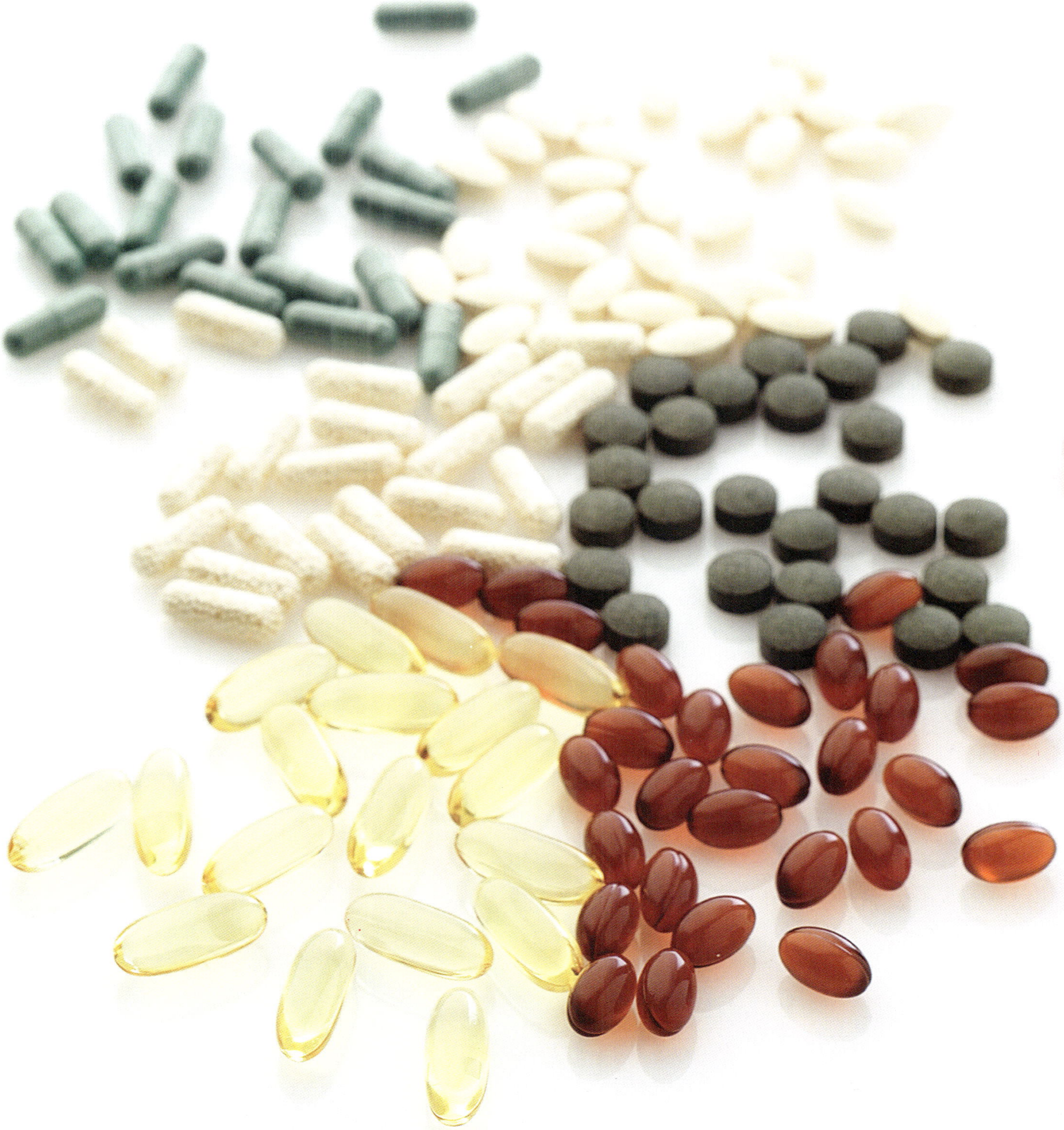

NUTRIENTS AND THEIR RICH FOOD SOURCES	
Vitamin A / Beta-carotene	Apricots, asparagus, broccoli, cantaloupe melon, carrots, collard greens, liver, pumpkin, spinach, sweet potatoes, watermelon
Vitamin D (cholecalciferol)	Cod liver oil, herring, mackerel, salmon, sardines
Vitamin E (alpha tocopherol)	Almonds, corn oil, filberts, sunflower seeds and oil, walnuts, wheatgerm, wholewheat flour
Vitamin C (ascorbic acid)	Blackcurrants, broccoli, Brussels sprouts, cabbage, collard greens, grapefruit, green peppers, guava, lemons, oranges, papaya, potatoes, spinach, strawberries, tomatoes, watercress
Vitamin B1 (thiamine)	Beef kidney and liver, brewer's yeast, brown rice, garbanzo beans, kidney beans, pork, rice bran, salmon, soybeans, sunflower seeds, wheatgerm, wholegrain wheat and rye
Vitamin B2 (riboflavin)	Almonds, brewer's yeast, cheese, chicken, mushrooms, wheatgerm
Vitamin B3 (niacin)	Beef liver, brewer's yeast, chicken, eggs, fish, sunflower seeds, turkey
Vitamin B5 (pantothenic acid)	Blue cheese, brewer's yeast, carrots, corn, eggs, lentils, liver, lobster, meats, peanuts, peas, soybeans, sunflower seeds, wheatgerm, wholegrain products
Vitamin B6 (pyridoxine)	Avocados, bananas, bran, brewer's yeast, carrots, filberts, lentils, rice, salmon, shrimps, soybeans, sunflower seeds, tuna, walnuts, wheatgerm, wholegrain flour
Vitamin B12 (cyanocobalamin)	Cheese, clams, eggs, fish, meat, milk and milk products
Antioxidants	Avocado, beets, berries, broccoli, cabbage, carrots, collard greens, fish, garlic, grapes, green tea, nuts, onions, peppers, prunes, raisins, seeds, sweet potatoes, tomatoes, watercress, wheatgerm
Biotin	Brewer's yeast, brown rice, cashew nuts, cheese, chicken, eggs, lentils, mackerel, meat, milk, oats, peanuts, peas, soybeans, sunflower seeds, tuna, walnuts
Calcium	Almonds, Brazil nuts, cheese, kelp, milk, molasses, salmon (canned), sardines (canned), shrimp, soybeans, yogurt
Carbohydrates	Bread, corn, crackers, noodles, oats, pasta, potatoes, rice, sweet potatoes
Chromium	Beef, brewer's yeast, chicken, eggs, fish, fruit, milk products, potatoes, whole grains

Coenzyme Q10	All foods, particularly, beef, mackerel, sardines, soy oil, spinach
Essential fatty acids (EFAs)	Fish (e.g. herring, mackerel, salmon, sardines, tuna); flaxseeds, pumpkin, sesame and sunflower seeds and their unprocessed oils
Fiber	Barley, beans (e.g. pinto, kidney, black-eyed, garbanzo), brown rice, buckwheat, fresh fruit, fresh vegetables, lentils, oats, rye, wholewheat
Folic acid	Barley, brewer's yeast, fruits, garbanzo beans, green leafy vegetables, lentils, peas, rice, soybeans, whole wheat, wheatgerm
Iodine	Cod-liver oil, fish, oysters, table salt (iodized), seaweed, sunflower seeds
Iron	Cashew nuts, cheese, egg yolk, garbanzo beans, lentils, molasses, mussels, pumpkin seeds, seaweed, walnuts, wheatgerm, whole grains
Magnesium	Almonds, fish, green leafy vegetables, kelp, molasses, nuts, soybeans, sunflower seeds, wheatgerm
Manganese	Avocados, barley, blackberries, buckwheat, chestnuts, filberts, ginger, oats, peas, pecans, seaweed, spinach
Potassium	Avocados, bananas, citrus fruits, lentils, milk, molasses, nuts, parsnips, potatoes, raisins, sardines (canned), spinach, whole grains
Protein	Dairy products, eggs, fish, meat, poultry, soy
Selenium	Broccoli, cabbage, celery, chicken, egg yolk, garlic, liver, milk, mushrooms, onions, seafood, wheatgerm, whole grains
Sodium	Bacon, bread, butter, canned vegetables, ham, milk, table salt and most commercially processed and packaged foods
Sulfur	Cabbage, clams, eggs, fish, garlic, milk, onions, wheatgerm
Zinc	Egg yolk, fish, all meat, milk, molasses, oysters, sesame seeds, soybeans, sunflower seeds, turkey, wheatgerm, whole grains

Although this book focuses primarily on the nutritional aspects of improving mood, many other forms of therapy can make a significant difference to how you feel. Looking after your body and mind should be a holistic experience that encompasses all aspects of what it is to be human.

feel good strategies

A healthy, balanced diet is a great starting point from which to address any mood-related problems you may be experiencing. However, your strategies for feeling better should not be limited to dietary changes. There are a host of additional ways of boosting your moods that involve looking beyond your body's nutritional needs. For example, appropriate, regular exercise can have a profound, long-lasting positive effect on your physical and emotional well-being. Similarly, sharing problems with a family member, friend, or professional therapist often leaves you feeling lighter and more at ease with yourself. You may choose to try one of the wide range of complementary therapies that can ease physical and mental symptoms, and also help you to relax and rediscover harmony between your body and mind. The alternative therapies covered here include acupuncture, homoeopathy, herbal medicine, flower essences, aromatherapy, and massage (see also Further Reading, page 138).

GET MOVING

Consider that one way of looking at low moods and fatigue is as negative energy in your body and mind, dragging you down. If you exercise, you are taking that negative energy and transforming it into a positive, life-enhancing force. However you choose to look at it, there is no getting away from the fact that exercise does make you feel better. Any lifestyle aimed at getting or maintaining a healthy body and mind must involve some sort of regular physical activity. It is something all of us are aware of, some of us do without fail, some of us get round to intermittently (and then remember how great it feels), and some of us ignore completely. Unless you are in the first category and therefore need no encouragement at all, the key to incorporating regular exercise into your weekly routine is to choose a form of physical activity that stimulates you, one you enjoy, and one that is appropriate for your level of strength and fitness.

Countless scientific studies have found that regular exercise can help maintain good moods and ultimately boost energy. Although the exact mechanism by which this works is not yet well understood, it is believed that exercise promotes the release of mood-improving chemicals—such as endorphins, norepinephrine (which is linked to improving drive and motivation), and even serotonin. These chemicals do not only give you a boost during your actual workout, but for some time afterward as well. Exercise also increases the supply of oxygen to every part of the body, which means that each cell is being better nourished and cleansed, enabling it to do its job optimally. Higher levels of oxygen stimulate your mind, too, allowing you to focus on your movements or breathing in an almost meditative way. Provided it is not too strenuous, exercise also improves immunity and helps reduce levels of cortisol (the stress hormone that in excess can leave you feeling exhausted, see page 20). On a psychological level, exercise often helps make you feel that you have achieved something positive, and provides a pleasant sense of personal accomplishment.

Exercise may consist of very simple activities, even just stretching at home. If you are unfit, suddenly going to the

TIPS FOR GETTING MOVING

The first step in beginning an exercise program is the all-important decision to get moving. Once you are feeling motivated you will be keen to discover and enjoy the benefits that exercise can bring. Bear these tips in mind, make sure you are well prepared, and go for it!

- Check with your doctor first if you have any doubt about your ability to exercise, for example if you have reason to be worried about your cardiac health, or suffer from any bone or muscle problems.
- Always start gently and build up slowly. If you are exercising at a club or in a class, talk to your trainer or teacher about what is best for you.
- Exercise at the time of day that feels right for you—there's no point in dragging yourself out of bed 90 minutes earlier than usual if it is just going to make you feel more exhausted and miserable. For many people, exercising toward the end of the day (but not too late in the evening) is best.
- Ideally, after eating, you should wait for two hours before exercising.
- Even if it is hard to get yourself going, it is important that you actually want to exercise, so choose an activity that inspires you and surround it with motivating add-ons, such as music and wearing comfortable, appropriate clothing/shoes.
- Exercising with a friend can help to motivate you.
- Exercise need not be fancy and expensive and require special gear. Even walking can be an excellent form of exercise: You can do it anywhere and it's free. Walking for just 20 minutes a day can make a difference. You could even incorporate it in your journey to work, your lunch break, or going to pick up the children from school. Make sure you walk in a safe area that is well lit if you walk at night.

gym and spending 45 minutes on the treadmill, even if you could manage it, would not be the best thing for you. In fact, your body would probably feel quite distressed. It is therefore very important to choose a form of exercise that is appropriate for you—it should be something that you will enjoy, the prospect of which is going to encourage you (at least most of the time), and which is not going to feel like a chore. Pushing yourself too hard is not helpful and may ultimately make you feel worse (studies have shown that even in very fit athletes, over-training can bring on depression and exhaustion). Start with a gentle activity, such as swimming or running, or perhaps take up a one-on-one game, such as badminton or tennis. Consider joining a team (as long as the level is appropriate to you)—playing a team sport, even once a week, can really make you feel like part of a network. On the other hand, you may be happiest going for a brisk walk by yourself or with your dog. Listening to music while you exercise—be it energizing or relaxing—can also contribute to the benefits if it means that you enjoy the experience more. Basically, go for whatever suits you.

Unfortunately, when you are feeling low emotionally you often lack the motivation to exercise (let's face it, even many people who are not depressed find it difficult to bring themselves to partake in some physical activity). In such a case, you may find it helpful to arrange to exercise with a friend, so that you can encourage one another.

Once you have started to exercise, even if it has involved a great deal of effort to get there, the benefits you will feel are likely to act as an incentive for you to make it a regular event. Don't give up if it is tough at first—often you have to almost force yourself to get started, in order to break the cycle of lethargy, but only then will the feeling of improved mood and higher energy come.

There are several forms of exercise which, although not directly considered aerobic, provide a remarkably good workout for the body at the same time as relaxing the mind. Most of these come from Eastern traditions—they include yoga or any of the martial arts-based forms, such as T'ai Chi. At the same time as invigorating your body, they can calm your mind in a powerful, meditative way.

TALK IT THROUGH

The old saying "a problem shared is a problem halved," like many such adages, has more than a grain of truth in it. If there is something playing on your mind, getting it out of your own head can often do wonders to dissipate the negativity it can create.

Sometimes it can really help to turn to a partner, friend, or co-worker to externalize a persistent thought, worry or concern—in doing so, you often obtain a broader perspective or an alternative viewpoint that helps to make the problem easier to cope with. However, at other times, you may feel that it would be easier to talk your worries through with a virtual stranger, someone more removed from your life, in which case seeking support from a professional therapist (see below) or life coach (see box, right) may be more useful. Either way, taking the step of admitting that you need support is often the highest hurdle to overcome. It can be very empowering to realize that reaching out for help is not only a sign of strength, but also a very normal, healthy human reaction.

Bridging the gap

Because low moods are very often precipitated by low self-esteem, a traumatic event, chronic stress in domestic or working life, repeated destructive behavioral patterns, or internalized anger, it is usually very helpful to break such patterns, to learn to deal with certain situations, or to learn to accept oneself. After all, life is always going to present us with difficulties, and it is how we perceive these and how we handle them that makes the difference. Talking therapies, such as counseling or some sort of psychotherapy, can be extremely useful in such situations. If you embark on such a program, bear in mind that therapy does not offer a "cure," is not always easy, and often involves a long-term investment of time and effort. However, your therapist can lend a non-judgmental, listening ear along the journey and the rewards, in terms of your emotional wellbeing, can be considerable.

Many scientific trials have tested the efficacy of various talking therapies compared with antidepressant medication. Several of these studies have shown cognitive therapy, for example, to be more effective than medication, while others have suggested that cognitive therapy adds to the efficacy of drug treatment. (Cognitive therapy addresses the cognitions—perception, intuition, reactions—that mediate the impact of events in a person's life.) I do not know of any trials comparing nutrient therapy with psychotherapy, but the studies do indicate that dealing with mood problems using any sort of physiological therapy (be it drugs or nutrition) is not the absolute answer to treating depression, and that psychotherapy can play an important role.

Exploring acceptance, self-worth, and how one deals with life events can be invaluable in overcoming persistent or recurring low moods or depression. Even if all biochemical imbalances are corrected, the mind's delicate equilibrium can be easily upset by negative behavioral patterns and reaction to stressors (see page 18).

LIFE COACHING

If the thought of entering into a therapy program of any sort does not appeal, perhaps life coaching would be more appropriate for you. Working with a life coach can give you the confidence and ability to move forward in the areas of your life where you feel you are in a rut. Life coaches recognize that it is often our own frustrations and sense of stagnation, along with our failure to realize our own potential, that can leave us feeling low. A professional life coach, who can often provide sessions by telephone or email, can help you in a variety of ways. He or she may:

- show you how to set more appropriate, realistic goals and then reach them
- encourage you to achieve more by working on ways to take down the barriers to doing so
- help you to focus better, to produce results more efficiently
- provide you with the tools, support, and structure to improve any area of your life

There are countless types of psychotherapy to choose from, but it appears that it is not the particular school of training that makes the most difference, but the strength of the bond between the therapist and client.

OTHER APPROACHES

For many of us with busy lifestyles, making time for ourselves is surprisingly difficult, and it is often something we relegate to the bottom of our list of priorities. However, "me time" is crucial to balancing everything else that is going on in our lives.

When you are feeling down, there are countless simple ways that you can give yourself a boost. Just taking some time out from your daily routine to relax and rejuvenate your body and mind—whether that be in the form of having a bath, playing with the children, or doing some exercise—can make a tremendous difference.

If you have been feeling persistently low for a long time, in addition to adopting the nutritional strategies described in this book, you may also want to try a complementary therapy that addresses stress-related problems and helps you to rediscover harmony between your body and mind. With the recent emergence of more and more variations of all sorts of therapies, there are plenty to choose from. Some of the most beneficial that I know of, or have experienced myself, are listed below.

Acupuncture

This is the ancient Eastern art of using very fine needles, which are painlessly inserted into special points along meridians (energy lines) in the body, to gently correct imbalances in the body's natural energy flow. A very powerful treatment, acupuncture can help deal with both physical and mental conditions. Scientific trials have found acupuncture to be at least as effective as drug therapy in combating depression.

Homoeopathy

This is one of the truly holistic therapies that, although seemingly incredibly subtle, can have remarkable effects. You are given a specifically chosen remedy by your homoeopath—in an infinitesimal dosage—which stimulates the body to heal any imbalances.

Herbal Medicine

Both the traditional Chinese and Western use of plants for medical purposes are almost as old as humankind itself. In the West, the best-known herb for helping balance mood is St John's Wort, which is among the most widely prescribed antidepressants in Germany. It is believed to work by increasing the levels of serotonin in circulation in the body. It is best to visit a qualified medical herbalist who can give you a prescription of this, or other herbs tailored to your personal needs.

Flower Essences

I have personally experienced remarkable benefits from using Australian Bush Flower Essences, although there are several others on the market, including the excellent Bach Flower Remedies. These essences are another very subtle but effective way of correcting all sorts of emotional imbalances. You can buy flower essences at most healthfood stores and pharmacists, and there are several books available that can help you choose which essences would be most appropriate for you (see page 138). However, like herbal remedies, flower essences are best taken under the guidance of an experienced healthcare practitioner.

Aromatherapy

The concentrated essential oils of plants are used for massage, inhalation, compresses, baths, and in special burners. When chosen by a trained aromatherapist, the blend of oils used can help to relieve a range of both emotional and physical conditions.

Massage

There are many types of massage available—from aromatherapy to deep-tissue to shiatsu. The best way to find out which is suited to you is to contact a local natural health clinic and discuss your wants and needs. When performed by a skilled practitioner, massage can have very profound physical and emotional effects.

glossary

Acetylcholine

The main **neurotransmitter** for communication between brain **neurons** that are responsible for, among other things, memory and cognitive thinking.

Epinephrine

Also known as adrenalin, this hormone is secreted by the adrenal glands as part of the body's response to stress. Epinephrine plays a role in effecting physiological changes that include faster breathing, raised heart rate, and increased levels of blood **glucose**, all of which are intended to enable the body to respond effectively to a stressful situation.

Amino acid

A building block of **protein**. All the proteins in the body are made up of combinations of any number of amino acids, of which there are about twenty in total.

Antioxidant

A substance—nutrient or enzyme—which can "disarm" an **oxidant**. In other words, antioxidants neutralize the potentially damaging effects of oxidation. Key antioxidant **nutrients** are vitamins A, C, and E. Fresh fruit and vegetables, nuts, seeds, and whole grains are all particularly rich sources of antioxidants.

Carbohydrate

A sugar or starch which is used by the body primarily as fuel for energy production. Rice, pasta, bread, potatoes, and sugar are rich sources of carbohydrates.

Cortisol

A hormone secreted by the adrenal glands in response to stress. Cortisol plays a part in effecting the physiologial changes that help the body deal with the stress, perceived or real. One of cortisol's key roles is to increase the supply of **glucose** to the brain and other tissues. Cortisol helps reduce inflammation, but also appears to interfere with the levels of the mood-boosting **neurotransmitters serotonin** and **dopamine** that the body produces.

DHA

DHA, or docosahexaenoic acid, is an **essential fatty acid** which is found in fish, and can also be produced in the body from fats contained in flaxseeds, hemp seeds, and walnuts. DHA is used in the body in the lining of nerves and cell membranes.

Dopamine

Like **serotonin**, dopamine is a **neurotransmitter** involved in mood and motivation. Dopamine can be made in the body from the **amino acids** phenylalanine and tyrosine.

EPA

EPA, or eicosapentaenoic acid, is an **essential fatty acid** that is in the same "family" as **DHA**. EPA is found in fish, and can also be made in the body from fats contained in flaxseeds, hemp seeds, and walnuts. EPA has many uses in the body, including forming part of the lining of nerves and cell membranes.

Essential fatty acids (EFAs)

A group of fats (oils) essential for many vital functions in the body, including healthy brain and nerve cells, balanced hormones, energy production, and well-hydrated skin. EFAs can only be obtained from the diet; rich sources are nuts, seeds, and oily fish.

Glucose

A type of sugar which is the prime source of fuel for energy in the brain as well as the rest of the body. The body converts **carbohydrates** into sugars such as glucose during the digestive process.

Gluten

A **protein** found in grains such as wheat, oats, rye, and barley.

Glycaemic index

A scale that measures the rate at which a particular food is digested and released as **glucose** into the blood stream. The faster a food raises blood-sugar levels, the higher it is rated on the GI scale.

Neuron

A nerve cell, sometimes called a neurone. Nerve cells exist throughout the body and brain.

Neurotransmitter

A chemical in the body which facilitates the transmission of impulses (messages) through the nervous system, from one **neuron** to the next.

Nutrients

All chemical reactions that take place in the body depend on a regular supply of "micro" nutrients, such as vitamins and minerals, and "macro" nutrients, including **protein**, **carbohydrates**, fats, and water.

Oxidants

Molecules that are by-products of oxygen and can be likened to "sparks" from anything that burns, including cigarettes and food, as well as the combustion of **glucose** in our cells to make energy. Oxidants can damage cells, thereby accelerating ageing and causing disease. **Antioxidants** help counter such damage.

Phosphatidyl choline (PC)

A type of **phospholipid** containing choline, which is incorporated into healthy cell membranes and needed to make **acetylcholine**. PC is also contained in bile where it contributes to the proper digestion of fats. Lecithin (found in soy, eggs, and as a food supplement) is a source of PC.

Phosphatidyl serine (PS)

A type of **phospholipid** that is an essential component of human cell membranes. PS, which is thought to play an important role in the body's **neurotransmitter** function, is found in small amounts in soy lecithin and is also available as a food supplement.

Phospholipid

A substance made of phosphorus and lipids (fats), phospholipid forms an important part of human cell membranes, including those of **neurons**.

Probiotics

A term used to describe the so-called "bacteria", such as Lactobacillus acidophilus and bifido bacteria, that are needed for healthy digestion. Probiotics are available as food supplements and are also found in live, natural yogurt.

Protein

Made of **amino acids**, proteins are used in the body to form the main structures, including all cells, as well as enzymes, hormones, and **neurotransmitters**. Fish, poultry, meat, milk, yogurt, cheese, and beans such as soy are rich sources of protein.

Saturated fat

A type of fat found mainly in animal-derived foods such as meat and dairy products. Saturated fats are not essential for human health and should not be consumed in large quantities.

Serotonin

A mood-boosting **neurotransmitter** that is involved in numerous processes in the body, including sending out the signals that control appetite. Serotonin is derived from the **amino acid tryptophan**.

Transfatty acid

A type of fat that has been transformed by exposure to excess heat or light, changing its chemical structure and rendering it harmful to the body. **EFAs** are particularly susceptible to oxidation damage, which can turn them into transfatty acids. Many commercially produced oils contain transfatty acids.

Tryptophan

An **amino acid** which is particularly abundant in bananas, chicken, figs, milk, seaweeds, sunflower seeds, tuna, turkey, and yogurt. Tryptophan can be converted in the body into the **neurotransmitter serotonin**.

Unsaturated fat

Considered to be far more healthy than **saturated fats**, unsaturated fats are found in vegetable sources, including oils such as olive, sunflower, safflower, rapeseed, soy, peanut, and sesame. Unsaturated fats can be further subdivided into monounsaturated and poly-unsaturated fats (the latter is another name for **essential fatty acids**).

further reading

Brewer, Dr Sarah *Simply Relax*, Duncan Baird Publishers, London (UK) and Ulysses Press, Berkeley, CA (US), 2000

Clayton, Paul *Health Defence*, Accelerated Learning Systems, Aylesbury (UK), 2001

Cousin, Pierre Jean *Food Is Medicine* (UK) / *Eat Well Be Well* (US), Duncan Baird Publishers, London (UK) and Thorsons, London (US), 2001

Erasmus, Udo *Fats that Heal, Fats that Kill*, Alive Books, Canada (UK and US), 1999

Geary, Amanda *The Food and Mood Handbook*, Thorsons, London (UK), 2001

George, Mike *Discover Inner Peace*, Duncan Baird Publishers, London (UK), 2000

Glenville, Marilyn *Natural Alternatives to HRT*, Kyle Cathie, London (UK) and Celestial Arts, Berkeley, CA (US), 1997

Hartvig, Kirsten *Eat for Immunity* (UK) / *Star Foods for Healthy Eating* (US), Duncan Baird Publishers, London (UK) and Thorsons, London (US), 2002

Holford, Patrick *Beat Stress & Fatigue*, Piatkus, London (UK), 1999

Holford, Patrick *6 Weeks to Superhealth*, Piatkus, London (UK), 2000

Idzikowski, Chris *Learn to Sleep Well*, Duncan Baird Publishers, London (UK) and Chronicle Books, San Francisco, CA (US), 2000

Jonsson, Gudrun *Gut Reaction*, Vermilion, London (UK) and Trafalgar Square, Vermont (US), 1999

Leeds, Dr Anthony et al. *The GI Factor*, Hodder & Stoughton, London (UK), 1996

Murray, Michael *The Healing Power of Herbs*, Prima Publishing, Roseville, CA (US, also UK), 1995

Philipott, William H. and Kalita, Dwight K. *Brain Allergies*, Keats Publishing, New Canaan, CT (UK) and McGraw-Hill, New York (US), 1987

Rowley, Nic and Hartvig, Kirsten *Detox for Health*, Duncan Baird Publishers, London (UK) and Thorsons, London (US), 2001

Rowley, Nic and Hartvig, Kirsten *Energize Your Life*, Thorsons, London (US), 2002

Rowley, Nic and Hartvig, Kirsten *Energy Foods*, Duncan Baird Publishers, London (UK), 2000

Rowley, Nic and Hartvig, Kirsten *Energy Juices*, Duncan Baird Publishers, London (UK), 2000

Scheffer, Mechthild *Bach Flower Therapy*, HarperCollins, London (UK) and Inner Traditions Intl Ltd (US), 1988

Schmidt, Michael *Smart Fats*, Frog Ltd, CA (UK and US), 1997

Smith, Karen *Massage*, Duncan Baird Publishers, London (UK) and John Wiley and Sons, New York (US), 1999

White, Ian *Bush Flower Essences*, Findhorn Press, Forres, UK and Tallahassee, FL (US), 1997

Worwood, Valerie *The Fragrant Pharmacy*, Bantam Books (UK) and Books Britain (US), 1991

Young, Jacqueline *Eastern Healing* (UK) / *The Healing Path* (US), Duncan Baird Publishers, London (UK) and Thorsons, London (US), 2001

Carol Vorderman's Detox for Life, Virgin, London (UK), 2001

useful addresses

For information about Natalie Savona, visit: www.nataliesavona.com

Institute for Optimum Nutrition

For details on ION courses and publications, visit: www.ion.ac.uk.

NOTE: The organizations listed below are entirely independent and are in no way connected to the information or recommendations in this book. To find out about psychotherapy or counseling, your first port of call could be your doctor, or ask friends to recommend someone. For information on yoga, t'ai chi, massage, aromatherapy, or other relaxation therapies, ask at your local natural health center or sports center.

In the UK:

UK Council for Psychotherapy

167–169 Great Portland Street
London W1W 5PF
Tel: 00 44 20 7436 3002
www.psychotherapy.org.uk
Email: ukcp@psychotherapy.org.uk

British Association of Counselling and Psychotherapists

1 Regent's Place
Rugby CV21 2PJ
Warwickshire
Tel: 00 44 1788 578 328
www.bac.co.uk

Women's Nutritional Advisory Service (WNAS)

www.wnas.org.uk

British Allergy Foundation

Deepdene House
30 Bellegrove Road
Welling DA16 3PY
Kent
Tel: 00 44 20 8303 8583
www.allergyfoundation.com

Eating Disorders Association

First Floor
Wensum House
103 Prince of Wales Road
Norwich NR1 1DW
Helpline: 00 44 1603 621 414
Administration: 00 44 870 770 3256
www.edauk.com

The Society of Homeopaths

4a Artizan Road
Northampton NN1 4HU
Tel: 00 44 1604 621400
www.homeopathy-soh.org/
Email: info@homeopathy-soh.org

In the US:

Eating Disorders Awareness and Prevention, Inc.

A non-profit organization devoted to the awareness and prevention of eating disorders:
http://www.edap.org/

For all types of information about eating disorders, visit this website:
http://www.something-fishy.org

Bastyr Naturopathic University

14500 Juanita Drive North East
Bothell
WA 98011
Tel: 425-823-1300
www.bastyr.edu

The American Association of Naturopathic Physicians

Suite 300
8201 Greensboro Drive
McLean
VA 22102
www.naturopathic.org

American Holistic Medical Association

6728 McLean Village Drive
McLean
VA 22101-8729
www.holisticmedicine.org

In Canada:

The Canadian Naturopathic Association (CNA)

1255 Sheppard Ave. East
North York
Ontario
M2K 1E2
Tel: 416-496-8633
www.naturopathicassoc.ca

index

Page numbers in *italics* refer to recipes incorporating particular foods.

A

acupuncture 135
addiction 39, 47, 61
adrenal glands
  blood-sugar balance 18, 20
  nutrients 17, 21
age-related cognitive decline (ARCD) 62
alcohol
  avoiding 30, 46, 57, 74
  blood-sugar balance 14, 69
  depression 69
alfalfa 51, *86*, *114*
allergens 38, 39, 76
allergies 38
almonds *122*
Antarctic icefish 76, *106*
anti-nutrients 25, 47, 128
antioxidants 29, 33–4, 65, 130
apples 32, 51, *82*, *121*
apricots *83*, *118*, *122*
aromatherapy 135
artichokes *91*
asparagus *83*
avocados *86*, *87*
avoidance testing 39

B

B vitamins
  blood-sugar balance 17
  brain 62, 65
  depression 22, 68, 69
  energy 46
bacteria 34–5
bananas 53, 56, 70, *121*
barley 34, *83*
basil 51, 79, *93*
bean sprouts *106*
beans 34, 51
  canned *89*, *91*, *98*, *113*
  runner *89*, *97*, *98*, *116*
  sprouted mung *114*
beetroot 65, *91*, *117*
berries 65, *83*, *121*
binge-eating disorder (BED) 58–61
black-eyed beans 34
blood-sugar balance 12–17, 74
  mood 18, 20–1, 50, 53, 61, 68–9
  nutrients 13, 17, 21, 24
borage 18, 26, 28
borlotti beans 34, *89*
bowels 33
brain
  choline 64
  fatty acids 28, 62, 68
  fuel 12, 14
  slow-down 62–5
  toxins 33
breakfasts 12, 16, 80–3
  balanced 44, 61, 80
broccoli *114*
brown rice 14, 34, 46, 78, *88*, *100*, *109*
buckwheat 34, *83*
butternut pumpkin *117*

C

cabbage
  red *84*, *90*
  white *114*, *116*
caffeine 46, 47
calcium 32, 57, 130
capers *102*
carbohydrates 130
  blood sugar 12, 14
  mood 70
  SAD 52–3
cardamom *118*
cardiovascular disease 65
carrots 51, *84*, *94*, *116*
cashew nuts *116*
cauliflower 64
celery 51, *94*
cell membranes 26, 65
chamomile 18, 57
cheese
  cottage *88*, *124*
  feta *90*, *100*
  goat's *84*, *100*, *124*
chemicals 51
chestnut mushrooms *80*, *87*
chicken 53, 56, 70, *84*, *86*, *87*, *106*, *110*
  stock *94*
chickpeas 34
chocolate 60, *118*
cholecystokinin (CCK) 60
choline 64
choosing food 77–9
chromium 17, 53, 61, 130
cigarettes 69, 74
citrus fruit 51
coconut milk 76, *96*
coffee
  avoiding 47, 57, 74, 79
  decaffeinated 47
  depression 69
cognitive therapy 134
complementary therapies 135
cooking oil 28, 76, 79
coriander 79, *116*

cortisol 20, 21, 54, 56, 69, 132
cottage cheese *88*, *124*
courgettes *98*, *100*, *102*, *113*
crackers, toppings *124*
cravings 17, 39, 50, 52–3, 58
crème fraîche *104*, *122*
crudités *124*
cucumber *92*, *114*

D

dehydration 44, 47
depression 66–71
  fatty acids 29
  SAD 52
  stress 20
desserts 118–23
detoxification 30–7, 71, 76
diet
  balanced 24–5
  blood-sugar balance 15
  detoxification 33, 36–7
  energy 45, 47
  "feel good" 74–7
  mood boost 71
  sleep 56
  stress 20–1
digestion 30–7, 76
dopamine
  mood 20, 53, 71
  nutrients 24, 53
dried fruit 15–16, *83*, *118*, *122*
drinks *see* coffee; juices; smoothies; tea; water
duck livers *91*

E

eating
  bingeing 58–61
  good habits 33, 60
eggplants *100*
eggs 46, 64, *80*, *83*, *88*, *100*, *118*
endorphins 60, 132
energy 44–7
  "drainers" 25, 47, 128
epinephrine 14, 18, 20, 21
essential fatty acids (EFAs) 26–9, 74, 76, 131
  brain 28, 62, 68
  stress 21
evening primrose oil 28
exercise 132–3
  adrenals 21
  depression 68
  detoxification 37

F

fats
  blood-sugar balance 17
  saturated 28, 76
  unsaturated 28
  see also essential fatty acids
fava beans *91*
"feel good" diet 74–7
fennel 51
feta cheese *90*, *100*
fiber 74, 131
  blood-sugar balance 17, 53
  detoxification 33, 34
  hormonal balance 50
figs 53, 56, 70
fish 46, 64
  oily 29, 68, 76, *87, 88, 92, 102, 105, 106, 109*
  stock *97*, *98*, *102*
  white *87, 97*, *102*, *104, 106*
flax *see* linseed
flower essences 135
folic acid
  depression 22
  food sources 131
food
  allergies 38
  cooking 25, 74
  frozen 25
  nutrients 130–1
  processed 15, 22, 25, 33
  sensitivities 38–9, 69
fruit
  canned *122*
  citrus 51
  dried 15–16, *83*, *118*, *122*
  fresh 34, 65, 66, 71, 74, *124*
  juices 15–16, 74, 79
  mixed *80*
  tropical *122*
  washing 78
  see also types of fruit

G

garlic 65, *90*, *109*, *110*, *113*
glucose
  brain fuel 12, 14
  energy 47
glycaemic index (GI) 16–17
goat's cheese *84*, *100*, *124*
green beans *89*, *97*, *98*, *116*
green vegetables 57

H

haddock *87*, *97*, *102*
hair-mineral analysis 32
haricot beans *98*
heart disease 28, 29
hemp seeds 26, 29
herbal medicine 135
herbs
  culinary 79
  infusions 57
  sedatives 57
  tea 18, 57, 79
  see also types of herbs

herring 29
High-Five Seeds *80*, *82*, *84*
homoeopathy 135
hops 57
hormonal balance 48–51
  depression 69
  fatty acids 28
  sleep 56
houmous 17, *86*
hydrogenated fat 29, 76

I

immunity 132
insomnia 54
insulin 15, 17
iron 44–5, 131

J

juices 15–16, 74, 79

K

key food groups 76–7
kidney beans 34

L

lamb *109*
  stock *98*
lecithin 64
leeks *80*, *94*, *97*
legumes 64
lemon balm 57
lentils 34, *90*, *93*, *110*
life coaching 134
light therapy 53
lima beans *98*
linseed 26, 29, 37, 51
linseed oil 29
liquorice 51
liver
  "flush" 37
  hormones 48, 50
  toxins 30, 32–3, 35
livers, duck *91*
lunches 84–93
lymphatic flow 37

M

mackerel 29, *87*, *105*, *109*
macro-nutrients 25
magnesium 17, 24, 50, 57, 131
main meals 100–13
manganese 17, 131
mangetout *84*, *106*
massage 135
meals
  balanced 24, 76
  regular 16, 21, 53, 66
meat, lean 46, 71
medication 46, 51, 71
memory decline 65
menopausal symptoms 51
metabolism 80
micro-nutrients 24, 47
milk 53, 56, 57, 64, 70, *118*
molasses 57
monkfish *97*, *102*
monounsaturated fats 28
muesli *121*
multivitamins 17, 50, 68, 70, 128
mung beans *114*
mushrooms
  chestnut *80*, *87*
  Portobello *113*
  shiitake *110*
  straw *98*
mussels *97*, *102*
myelin 62

N

nettles *105*
neurons 24, 62
neurotransmitters 62, 71
norepinephrine 132
nut butter *124*
nutrients 22–5
  adrenals 17, 21
  blood-sugar balance 13, 17, 21, 24
  detoxification 34
  digestion 34
  energy 45
  food sources 130–1
  mood 20, 68
  sleep 57
  see also anti-nutrients; key food groups
nutritional supplements 68, 69, 70, 128–9
  blood-sugar balance 17
  brain 62
  detoxification 37
  digestion 37
  energy 46, 47
  PMS 50
nutritionists 25, 35, 128
nuts 46, 57, 71, *124*
  almonds *122*
  cashew *116*
  pine *122*
  pistachio *118*

O

oats 34, 51, 57, *82*, *83*
oestrogen 48–51
oil
  cooking 28, 76, 79
  salad 78–9
  see also types of oil
olive oil 28, 78, *84*, *87*, *88*, *89*
omega-3 fats 26, 28–9, 62, 68
omega-6 fats 28–9, 68
onions 65, *88*, *90*, *113*
  spring *84*, *88*, *89*, *92*, *93*, *116*
organic produce 25, 78

overeating *see* binge-eating disorder (BED)
oxidants 33, 65
oxygen 65, 132

P
papaya, green *116*
parsley 51, *87*, *114*
passionflower 57
peaches *118*
pears 51, *118*, *122*
peas 51
  mangetout *84, 106*
pellagra 22
peppers
  green *88*, *113*
  red *87*, *88*, *91*, *102*, *113*
  yellow *102*
phototherapy 53
phyto-oestrogens 51
pilchards 29
pine nuts *122*
pineapple *122*
pinto beans 34, *89*
pistachio nuts *118*
poly-unsaturated fats *see* essential fatty acids
Portobello mushrooms *113*
potassium 79, 131
potatoes *86*, *97*, *100*, *109*
poultry 46
  see also chicken; turkey
premenstrual syndrome (PMS) 48–51, 56
probiotics 34–5
processed foods 15, 22, 25, 33
progesterone 48, 51
protein 74, 131
  blood sugar 16, 17, 21, 53, 80
prunes *122*
psychotherapy 134–5
pumpkin oil 78
pumpkin seeds 29, 79, *83*, *121*

Q
quinoa *113*, *114*

R
raisins *83*, *122*
rapeseed oil 28
raspberries *121*
recipes 80–125
red cabbage *84*, *90*
refined foods 46, 53, 74
rice
  bran 51
  brown 14, 34, 46, 78, *88*, *100*, *109*
  cakes 17
  noodles *84, 96*
  pancakes *106*
  wild *100*
runner beans *89*, *97*, *98*, *116*
rye 34, *83*
  bread *80*, *88*

S
sage 51
salad dressings 114
salad leaves *91*
salads 84, 88–93, 114–17
salmon 29, *87*, *102*, *106*
salt 48, 79
sardines 29
saturated fat 28, 76
scallops *102*
seafood 57
  see also mussels; prawns; scallops; shrimps; squid
seasonal affective disorder (SAD) 52–3, 58
seaweed 32, 53, 56, 70, 78, *116*
sedatives 57
seeds 29, 57, 65, 68, 71, 76, *124*
serotonin
  mood 20, 52–3, 61, 70, 71, 132
  nutrients 24, 53
  sleep 56
sesame 51
sesame seeds 29, 79, *106*
shiitake mushrooms *110*
shrimps *86, 96*, *97*, *98*, *102*, *104*
side dishes 114–17
sleep 37
  problems 54–7
smoking 69, 74
smoothies 79
snacks 124–5
  blood-sugar balance 61
  detoxification 37
  sleep 56
sodium 79, 131
soups 94–9
soy 51
  yogurt *80*
spice teas 79
spinach *84*, *110*, *114*
spring onions *84*, *88*, *89*, *92*, *93*, *116*
squash *117*
squid *102*, *110*
starches 14
starters 84–93
stimulants
  avoiding 25, 32–3, 47, 53
  blood sugar 14–15, 21, 53, 69
  depression 69, 71
  sleeplessness 56
straw mushrooms *98*
stress 18–21, 32
sugar
  avoiding 15, 61, 74
  foods containing 15–16
  mood 69

sunflower oil 28, 78
sunflower seeds 29, 46, 53, 56, 70, 79, *83*, *104*
sweet potato *91*, *117*
swordfish *102*

T

tamari 78
tea
  avoiding 74
  herbal 18, 57, 79
  spice 79
thyme 79
thyme oil 65
thyroid gland 45
tiredness 44–5
tomatoes *88*, *89*, *91*, *93*, *102*, *114*
  canned *90*, *102*, *109*
  cherry *84*, *92*, *109*, *113*, *116*
toppings
  baked potatoes 86–7
  crackers *124*
toxins 32–3, 35, 69, 71
trans-fats 29
triglycerides 28, 68
tropical fruit *122*
trout, rainbow *104*
tryptophan 53, 56, 61, 70
tuna 53, 56, 70
  canned *87*, *88*
  fresh 29, *92*
turkey 53, 56, 70, *100*, *109*
turmeric 78

U

unsaturated fat 28

V

valerian 57
vanadium 17
vegetables 25, 34, 65, 74
  cooking 25, 74
  fresh 34, 50, 71
  green 57
  stock *94*, *97*
  washing *78*
vitamins
  food sources 130
  requirements 24–5
  see also B vitamins

W

walnuts 29, *121*
water
  requirement 35, 74, 79
  retention problems 48
watercress *114*
wheat 38
wheatgerm 46, 51, *83*
white beans *91*
whole grains 46, 71
wild rice *100*

X

xeno-oestrogens 51

Y

yogurt 34–5, 53, 56, 70, *80*, *83*, *86*, *118*, *122*, *124*

Z

zinc 32, 131

acknowledgments

Thank You ... to Anne-Lise Miller for first opening my naive eyes to the connection between my body and my mind; to Patrick Holford for his ongoing inspiration about the power of good nutrition; to Judy Barratt, Joanne Clay, Manisha Patel, and the team at DBP for creating this beautiful book out of my words; to all those who contributed recipes; to Lisa Darnell for her priceless support; to Helen Bodger, Kate Cassidy, Susan Elderkin, Trisha Mulholland, Kate Rew, and Charmaine Yabsley for buoying me up; to Splash for being my playmate; to Amanda Bluglass for inspiring me to reach the finish line more quickly; to my parents, Joe and Joan, and my sister, Arielle for more love than anyone could ever wish for.